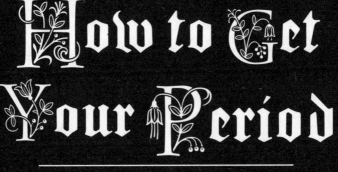

How to Get Your Period

A Guide to Performing Menstrual Extraction

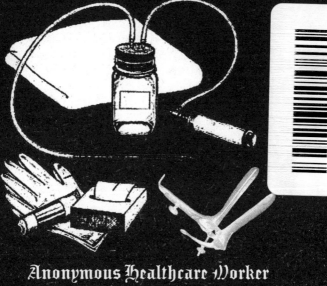

Anonymous Healthcare Worker

Microcosm Publishing

Portland, OR | Cleveland, OH

HOW TO GET YOUR PERIOD: A GUIDE TO MENSTRUAL EXTRACTION

ISBN 9781648413360
This is Microcosm #797
Second Edition, first published March 2024
This edition © Microcosm Publishing, 2022, 2024

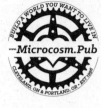

For a catalog, write or visit:
Microcosm Publishing
2752 N Williams Ave.
Portland, OR 97227

https://microcosm.pub/ME

To join the ranks of high-class stores that feature Microcosm titles, talk to your rep: In the U.S. *COMO* (Atlantic), *ABRAHAM* (Midwest), *BOB BARNETT* (Texas, Arkansas, Oklahoma, Louisiana), *IMPRINT* (Pacific), *TURNAROUND* (Europe), *UTP/MANDA* (Canada), *NEWSOUTH* (Australia/New Zealand), *OBSERVATOIRE* (Africa, Middle East, Europe), *Yvonne Chau* (Southeast Asia), *HARPERCOLLINS* (India), *EVEREST/B.K. Agency* (China), *TIM BURLAND* (Japan/Korea), and *FAIRE* and *EMERALD* in the gift trade.

Did you know that you can buy our books directly from us at sliding scale rates? Support a small, independent publisher and pay less than Amazon's price at **www.Microcosm.Pub**.

Global labor conditions are bad, and our roots in industrial Cleveland in the '70s and '80s made us appreciate the need to treat workers right. Therefore, our books are MADE IN THE USA.

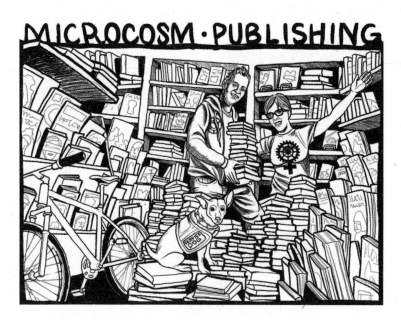

MICROCOSM PUBLISHING is Portland's most diversified publishing house and distributor, with a focus on the colorful, authentic, and empowering. Our books and zines have put your power in your hands since 1996, equipping readers to make positive changes in their lives and in the world around them. Microcosm emphasizes skill-building, showing hidden histories, and fostering creativity through challenging conventional publishing wisdom with books and bookettes about DIY skills, food, bicycling, gender, self-care, and social justice. What was once a distro and record label started by Joe Biel in a drafty bedroom was determined to be *Publishers Weekly*'s fastest-growing publisher of 2022 and #3 in 2023, and is now among the oldest independent publishing houses in Portland, OR, and Cleveland, OH. We are a politically moderate, centrist publisher in a world that has inched to the right for the past 80 years.

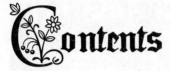

Contents

"What did women do before they had doctors? It can't be that hard. Let's just stop the frustration and humiliation of trying to persuade the powers that be to legalize abortion. Let's just take back the technology, the tools, the skills, and whatever else we need."

~Lorraine Rothman[1]

1 Chalker, R. and Downer, C. (1996) *The Woman's Book of Choices: Abortion, Menstrual Extraction, RU-486.* p.115

Introduction

eople all over the world have long sought access to affordable, legal, and humane reproductive health care. Since the mid-twentieth century in the United States, we have enjoyed a taste of reproductive freedoms offered by clinics and pharmacies. When the June, 2022 U.S. Supreme Court Dobbs v. Jackson Women's Health decision ended federal abortion protections offered by Roe v. Wade, a cascade of trigger laws were set into effect, immediately illegalizing abortion in numerous states and reducing access in others. Emboldened by the Dobbs decision, pro-life lobbies are proposing and passing law changes left and right, leaving us with confusing and unstable access to abortion care and paranoid about persecution. Soon even those of us who vote pro-life could lose reproductive and contraceptive health care provisions they had taken for granted.

We've had a taste of reproductive freedoms, and by no means will everyone be satisfied to stop seeking care and pushing for their rights. History informs us birth control and abortion attempts continue with or without government sanction. It's likely more people will return to using self-help methods conceived prior to Roe v. Wade, and underground networks will flourish. But how do we keep one another safe?

This book is intended to inform the reader about Menstrual Extraction (ME), a method of avoiding pregnancy which is safer, more accessible, and so far more legal than other notorious last resorts. Menstrual extraction is performed around the time of anticipated menstruation, by people trained inside a self-help network. This book is also intended to encourage the growth of self-help networks, such that basic reproductive care becomes available and affordable to more people.

What goes largely unsaid and misunderstood is the fact that working together, we still hold great agency over our reproductive health. We upkeep wisdom and safety in numbers. ME can't help us once our period is more than a couple weeks late, but it sure is a valuable tool to have in the toolbox in cases where birth control methods weren't used or available, or failed.

Hopefully the push to restore abortion rights will redouble as people come face-to-face with the realities of a pro-life state. Perhaps just as occurred in the 1970s, menstrual extraction will flourish and maybe even new methods of self-managed abortion will come to light. Meanwhile, let us take care of one another. We'll get through this.

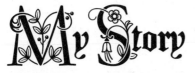

My Story

*T*first realized I was pregnant while floating in a pool in upstate New York. It just suddenly all came together: the nausea, fatigue, bloating, and *the unused pads in my purse.* Within hours, I had one hand on a positive pregnancy test stick and the other hand clutching my Aunt's voice, inside my first-ever cell phone. This was 1996. She said to travel east to where she was staying with friends and that she knew someone who could help me. I didn't know what other options I had since I was far away from home, and trusted her.

Before long I was being introduced to an older woman in the friends' driveway. She fished a medical duffel from her car trunk. Once inside, she and I were invited to use a quiet and dimly lit child's room. As instructed, I laid down on an absorbent pad set on a ruffly pink duvet amidst a sea of dolls and fluffy teddy bears.

Just like at the gynecologist's, I was asked questions about my cycle and contraception. Then I was gently asked to spread my legs, a speculum was inserted, and a relative stranger looked and poked inside me. She was reassuring and moved confidently, and soon enough I felt about as normal as if I was having a pedicure. Truly, the duvet and the dolls were the most awkward part: I was having an abortion in some little girl's room!

After swabbing my insides with antiseptic, the woman spent some time working a tube through my cervix. I cramped quite a bit. She then moved the tube slightly in and out after creating some suction on a small suction contraption. A tiny bit of blood sputtered into its jar. She seemed to be struggling to extract much blood, and eventually gave up. She was sweet and matter-of-fact when she said it may or may not have worked, but that I'd know soon. I remember thanking her as she placed her duffle back in her trunk and we gave her $75. Two hours later, while reading in bed and waiting for dinner, a torrent of blood gushed between my legs. The dinner bell rang. I was no longer pregnant.

I had a strong grasp on reproductive health at that point, but that experience was a blur. It didn't quite fit into what I knew. Here's what I knew: Nearly twenty years prior on a farm down the road, I was born on my parents' bed. My mother's midwife is legendary well beyond our family birth tales. I grew up wanting to do what she did. In high school, I wrote a 72-page essay on home birth. I learned I possessed agency over my body, and grew determined to control my own fertility. Even a mini-dose of the Pill gave me severe panic attacks, and cervical caps and diaphragms were too tricky for me to manage. I relied on condoms and the rhythm method, and so I suffered several pregnancy scares. This might sound strange, but even though I wanted to be a midwife, I did not want children.

I remember finding a copy of *Herbal Abortion,* a classic photocopied manifesto with a yarn-stitched spine, while working at Tower Books. I was still only a teenager, but knew well that herbs were medicine. It was wild to learn herbs could even be used as birth control and to induce menses, and that people could control their fertility, same as they could navigate their own childbirths.

Herbal wisdom from that book (along with other sources to corroborate it) helped me to bring on late periods several times. I certainly wasn't above putting parsley and garlic in my vagina! I even looked at my own cervix, something I'm pretty sure none of my buddies were doing. I thought I was pretty savvy! So it was just a surprise to meet a woman who did what I thought only doctors would do. I learned I had so much more agency with my own body.

My home abortion was unusual enough that I felt weird mentioning it, even with people I knew could understand. It's an almost unbelievable story, one that happened in a different dimension... surrounded by teddy bears and frilly pillows. I never regretted it and it didn't make me feel bad. My boyfriend wasn't happy, but was only able to vocalize being upset about helping me pay for it. I walked away feeling lucky to have had "as good an abortion as there was to be had."

What I regret is not telling more people about it, and not keeping in touch with that wonderful woman to learn more about her. Was she part of some network my aunt was tapped into?

Anyway, wherever you are, thank you.

A few years later, I studied to become a doula. On our first day of class we performed vaginal exams on one another on the floor of a conference room. "Wow, hi, nice to meet you!" It was incredible how I went from feeling horrified that everyone in the room would be stripping to the waist, to feeling like I was at the gynecologist with a very shy but gentle examiner, to sharing a really empowering breakthrough with that examiner. We looked at each other's nethers and the only reason it was a big deal was that we at least momentarily obliterated our self-consciousness and shame.

I pursued a career in midwifery as I had always longed to do, but grew profoundly disillusioned by medical management of childbirth while still in school attending hospital births. During that same time, I worked several weeks as an assistant at a busy clinic that provided abortions as well as comprehensive medical care. I learned in a general sense how the clinic operated. In reality, abortion didn't match what I saw in scary, bloody pro-life propaganda. I saw tears flow but also a lot of relieved smiles. Each night after shift came the scariest part: loaning courage to doctors by walking them to their cars. Births. Abortions. I wouldn't ever say these were opposite experiences or even on any spectrum; they are just part of our lives, and always will be.

Somehow I haven't bumped into anyone who spoke of knowledge of such a thing as "home abortion" since 1996, but I have learned through research that there is an underground network of people self-helping themselves to abortions and other gynecological care. They might call themselves part of the network, a self-help group, a friendship group, or another creative "team-like" name. One group, more focused on providing access to medicalized abortions in Chicago pre-Roe v. Wade, famously called themselves the Janes.[2] Over one hundred group members used the pseudonym Jane, such that if "Jane" called, you would probably know what it was about. They managed to help people obtain more than 11,000 safe first- and second-trimester abortions over four years[3]. All around the world, people gather to help one another, especially where medicine and/or the law fail them.

It turns out these networks shrank in America when abortion was legalized, to the point where maybe only a couple hundred members were active. How incredibly lucky I was to have met one of them. Now I listen amongst friends and acquaintances for any clue they might be familiar with any such network or willing to join. I built my suction contraption and do my own cervical exams. I'm ready and hope to help get you ready, too!

---

2 nytimes.com/2018/10/14/us/illegal-abortion-janes.html October 2018
3 Kaplan, L. (1995) *The Story of Jane: The Legendary Underground Feminist Abortion Service.*

How to Use This Book

So, you want to get your period. Maybe you have a big date, vacation, or wedding, and want to get the bleeding over with beforehand. Maybe you want to learn hands-on, in a supportive group, about your body and cycle.

Or maybe the stakes are higher. Almost anyone with a uterus has been there. We assumed our contraceptive would work. We thought we were sterile. We chose not to take the Plan B pill. Our condom broke. Darn it—we had already passed some points of turning back, and now we're worried we are pregnant! We are mostly sure we don't want to be pregnant, and that's enough surety. What are the options at this point?

Menstrual extraction (ME) is an option in all these scenarios. In the following pages I will introduce the history, art, and science of ME. We'll go over some basic anatomy and fertility concepts. Then we will work our way into some more advanced knowledge about menstrual extraction and how it could fit in your toolbox.

Finally, we'll talk about other options to explore if you are concerned you might be pregnant—or know that you are—and don't want to be.

It's best to study *How to Get Your Period* when you are not pregnant and prepare for a time in the future where you or someone you know needs help to bleed. Learn, plan, and find/form a network. If you are pregnant now and cannot find access to a self-help network, please keep reading through to the resources section at the end, and seek help through your medical provider or nearest legal abortion clinic.

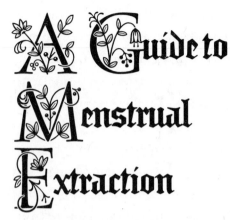

A Guide to Menstrual Extraction

Menstrual Extraction Is Born

n 1970, Carol Downer, a mother of six and a Los Angeles feminist activist, caught her first glimpse of a cervix during an IUD implantation. She was "bowled over" at how "simple and accessible our anatomy is."[4] Her life was essentially changed. Carol helped organize empowering self-help clinics, through which she met mother of four Lorraine Rothman. Rothman recalls Downer hopping up on a table at the first meeting and inserting a speculum in her vagina so that other self-help group members could see *just how accessible* it was. Downer's cervix has since become somewhat infamous, while she herself is an icon of women's rights activism.

---

4 *A Woman's Book of Choices* by Chalker and Downer, 1996, pg 114

Soon after, Rothman took it upon herself to improve upon a suction kit used by Harvey Karman, a Los Angeles layman who had been performing underground abortions safely for years.[5] Her contraption was very similar to Karman's, but included at least three improvements: adding a check valve to prevent air being pushed into the uterus, adding a jar to prevent uterine contents going directly and inconveniently into the vacuum syringe, and devising a setup that could be constructed at home by just about anyone. One aspect they readily adopted from Karman was the unpatented "Karman cannula" (CAN-you-la), a drinking straw-like tube used to pass through the cervix and siphon uterine contents. They liked that it was more flexible at the tip than other cannulas being used (specifically metal cannulas), and therefore less likely to perforate the uterus. Then and to this day, not just any plastic cannula will do. The Karman cannula has two large offset eyelets at the tip which prevent clogging. The eyelets tend to crease and fold if pressed with too much pressure, making the cannula much less likely to pierce body tissues.

5 Woo, E. (May 18 2008) *Creator of device for safer abortions.* LA Times latimes.com/archives/la-xpm-2008-may-18-me-karman18-story.html

Rothman and Downer knew they were onto something good. To be sure, they also took a field trip north to observe a Washington State abortionist practicing a more aggressive and painful style of abortion (D&C, dilation and curettage). The curettage, or "scraping" of the uterus, in D&C seemed overboard and unnecessarily painful to the two women. They were convinced their adapted vacuum kit would not only work, but be more accessible, more comfortable, and safer than vacuum kits used and documented since 1863. The duo had finally reclaimed abortion care from inventors and physicians who didn't need and would never have abortions, and delivered it generously into the hands of people who would.

Downer and Rothman dubbed what they planned to do "menstrual extraction" (ME) and named the menstrual extraction kit "Del-Em" in 1971. Rothman, wanting to keep the original meaning behind the cipher "Del-Em" as the dirty inside joke it once was in order to protect the dignity of menstrual extraction, will have you know that Del-Em stands for "Deliberate Emptying of Menses."[6]

6 Baumgardner, J. (2008) *Abortion & Life*, pg 25

Thanks to a spirited nationwide tour and relentless outreach, their self-help clinics spun off into splinter groups all over the United States, composed of people willing and able to perform not only self-exams, but safe and discreet menstrual extractions. Downer and Rothman delivered an even more accessible means for people to reclaim power over their health, cycles, and fertility.

In the United States, the 1973 Roe v. Wade decision confirmed the constitutional right to choose abortion. After several years of proselytizing self-help, menstrual extraction, and body empowerment, Carol Downer and Lorraine Rothman settled down and... opened a network of feminist, legal abortion clinics in California and beyond. The number of menstrual extractions performed in the United States began a decline. Menstrual extraction was certainly never less accessible or safe because of the Roe v. Wade ruling, so perhaps people just chose to exercise their federal rights and avoid the legal gray area self-managed abortion presents.

Is menstrual extraction legal? Probably not, but as of this writing nobody has ever been charged with a crime for extracting their period blood.

Every U.S. state has laws which *could* be used to prosecute someone who manages their own abortion.[7] If you are caught, how you've gone about things, whether or not a pregnancy was terminated, whether or not anybody was harmed, if the extractee is a minor, which state you are in, and how and where you are legally represented will all be factors in prosecution. One tradition in ME circles is to *not* take pregnancy tests before proceeding, and to *not* examine aspirated blood and tissue afterward. Remember menstrual extraction is just that – extraction of menses, not an abortion. Not having evidence of pregnancy provides some degree of deniability, meaning ME could be compared to common at home-procedures like self-catheterization, bladder irrigations... or the removal of menstrual blood. I cannot advise other than to say, yes, maybe don't have a witnessed pregnancy test, use ME as close to the anticipated date of menstruation as possible, definitely do not tell anyone you cannot absolutely trust, and consult with a lawyer about the gray areas. Study the skills and knowledge carefully and perform ME with capable, reliable help. And be aware that anti-choice lawmakers are more powerful and eager than ever to make a case.

---

7   ourbodiesourselves.org/2018/02/safe-and-supported-inside-the-diy-abortion-movement/

The Network of Self-Help Clinics

How do you find a self-help group in order to learn and carry out reproductive care and menstrual extraction? Perhaps you are only a degree of separation away through a doula or midwife friend, or an older friend who gave birth to many children, or perhaps another friend who has "seen and done it all" when it comes to holistic healing and alternative therapies. After calling down your phone list of most trusted buddies, we hope you are connected with someone in the network, or at least someone with some skills who is willing to help. It's possible you might have to travel to meet this person/group, or they will travel to meet you; either way, it's highly likely their time will cost you significantly less than a clinic visit.

Hopefully they make you feel comfortable about speaking frankly about things often considered shameful and secret. Things about your body and your life are not shameful and need not always be secret; in fact, we are 100% certain you will feel better getting it off your chest if you feel like it. No confidence in this person/group or feeling shady? Ask your questions because they are valuable, and trust your gut. Usually friends of friends are reliable, but that isn't always the case. Your health and sanity come first.

You may not need an abortion now or ever, nor may anyone you know, but statistically that is unlikely. Follow along and learn about menstrual extraction, and if anything, learn to do a self-exam and build a ME kit as a conversation piece for your next house party or show and tell. We need everyone to understand they have this option, whether it be to simply avoid having a period during a honeymoon or hot date, or to avoid being a parent when really not ready!

> *"...the most unsafe abortion is still safer than being forced to have a child, just to give you perspective."*
>
> *~Carol Downer at 88 years old[8]*

Safety Considerations

Menstrual extraction (ME) is a safe, non-medicalized home procedure that is widely used all over the world to remove menstrual blood through vacuum aspiration—essentially, suction. Menstrual extraction might be done to avoid having a menstrual period, to hurry along a heavy or painful period, or to avoid having a baby. Most ME providers prudently cut off at 6 weeks gestation, or when a period is two weeks late.

---

8 bitchmedia.org/article/Secret-Abortion-Body-Autonomy
January 2022

What makes menstrual extraction special is how accessible and safe it was designed to be. The supplies are (for the most part) easily sourced and the suction kit can be put together out of parts found at your local shops. Users are encouraged to become familiar with and unafraid of their anatomy, and realize this skill isn't much more complex than self-catheterization for urinary bladder problems. That said, it's nearly impossible to perform ME safely alone and/or without training. Menstrual extraction has never been a DIY thing, it's a do-it-together thing. Self-help groups form for the purpose of discussion and training around reproductive self-care, and the occasional practice of menstrual extraction. A circle is formed around the subject. And by nature of always having more eyes and hands on the subject, there is more compassion, perception, mutual understanding, and safety. Finally, the primary possible complication of ME (retained tissue) is resolved by simply repeating the ME procedure.

Because of the underground/private nature of ME, we won't find many reliable statistics about its use and safety. However, manual vacuum aspiration (MVA), a similar but medicalized precursor to ME, has been recorded in use since the early 1960s by the legitimized medical community. MVA is medicalized in the sense that you visit a licensed clinic for a MVA and typically a licensed or professionally-trained provider performs the aspiration. Sanctioned medical equipment, instruments, and sometimes also prescription medications are used. MVA providers usually have access to the cannulas, skills, and tools required and might evacuate advanced gestations beyond 6 weeks (but inside the first trimester).[9] MVA has caught on all over the globe and is endorsed by NGOs and governments because it is safe and effective.

In countries such as Bangladesh, Cuba, Korea, Singapore, Thailand, Hong Kong, and Vietnam, vacuum aspiration is commonplace and relatively shameless.[10] In those countries it is often called "menstrual regulation," possibly because it is more often performed without proof of pregnancy, and usually before a menstrual period is two weeks late. In other places, it might even be called a "mini-abortion" or "mini-suction."

The names seem somewhat interchangeable, but what sets menstrual extraction apart is the homemade Del-Em device used for the procedure, its fairly-secret network of people committed to cooperative self-help, and its non-medicalization.

---

9 The first trimester ends after gestational week 12, and the second trimester begins week 13.
10 en.wikipedia.org/wiki/Menstrual_extraction

A Del-Em is not an MVA kit. Most MVA kits are distributed by IPAS, an NGO dedicated to making abortion safe. ME and MVA are different mainly due to setting, and so even though you can learn a lot about ME by learning about MVA, keep them separate in your mind. Later I'll be explaining how to build a Del-Em and how one is used.

Risks and Cautions

This book was written by a medical professional who has experienced a menstrual extraction and witnessed home births, hospital births, and clinic abortions. This piece is not medical or legal advice and should not replace medical or legal advice, nor should anything in this piece be misconstrued as an endorsement of a technique or option.

Clinic-based health care comes with its risks as does home-based health care, and knowing what those risks and options are is a key part of being able to make good choices for your own health and to support others. We offer this information in the spirit of choice.

Finally, please do not attempt to do this alone, emotionally or physically. Ask for help. You will be surprised by the support and understanding you can find amongst trusted family and friends if you ask for help.

Do not attempt to freestyle, amend, or change the ME technique. The technique was honed in the 1970s and remains unchanged simply because it works. Know what you are doing, and be certain that what you're about to do has been done safely many times before.

The Importance of Gestational Age

A pregnancy test might confirm we are pregnant, but how far along are we? Sometimes we are asked what the first day of our last menstrual period (LMP) or last normal menstrual period (LNMP) was. Clinicians use this knowledge not just to gauge where we are in our menstrual cycle, but also to calculate gestational age if we might be pregnant. Knowing gestational age is crucial in determining appropriate pregnancy care, and also in choosing safe and appropriate abortion options.

Gestational age is usually the number of weeks since the first day of your LNMP. Keep in mind that gestational age is different from fetal age, because conception doesn't usually occur until two weeks after a LNMP. Despite this confusing little calendar knot, just remember: we measure gestational age forward in weeks from the first day of LNMP. I keep a handy gestation calculator or "pregnancy wheel" plastic dial in my medical kit, but I'm sure these days there's an app for that, too.

Not everyone has regular, "normal" periods or makes a good habit of tracking their periods, and some people spot at the beginning of pregnancy. So clinicians will often confirm gestational age using ultrasound. Those of us who can't do ultrasounds will just need to wrack brains and dig through memories. Will scrolling through photos on our phone remind us when we were last bleeding? Were we bleeding during a recent major holiday or party? Did we run out of period products and maybe have receipts for buying more? Try to guess within four days of the true date.

If it's still a riddle, stay in Sherlock Holmes mode until you have the best possible estimate of LNMP dates. Gestational age is a very important piece of data which we need to continue.

Reasons to Not Perform Menstrual Extraction
- IUD inside the uterus, suspected uterine deformity, or pelvic mass

- Abdominal or pelvic pain, known STD infection, pelvic inflammatory disease (PID), or fevers. Refer this person to a doctor.

- You do not have the correct instruments

- Anyone present is intoxicated

- Something doesn't feel right

- You or they don't want to continue

Health conditions such as asthma, epilepsy or heart problems could be exacerbated by the stress of ME. Proceed with caution and have a "what if" plan.

Always feel free to *not* continue, no matter what part of the process you've reached.

Risks of Menstrual Extraction

Cramping and blood loss due to ME can end pregnancy.

ME may fail to remove fetal tissue, i.e. "products of conception" (POC) if present. Here's the catch: the longer the gestation period, the easier it is to tell if the fetal sac has been removed. However, the longer the gestation period, the more inappropriate, difficult, uncomfortable and risky ME grows. Retained POC can be a breeding ground for bacterial overgrowth – bacteria which may otherwise normally live harmlessly inside the uterus.

Bacterial overgrowth or other germs introduced into the uterus could lead to pelvic infection and inflammation, which could cause permanent reproductive damage or death if untreated. Take extra special precaution in the presence of STD or if immunocompromised.

Perforation of the uterus or other internal organ could occur. This is rare: after following 10,000 cases of menstrual regulation (not ME) with appropriate instruments and technique, a study found that perforation occurred at a rate of 1:3500.[11] Perforation is more common when rigid cannulas are used. Uterine perforations which occur earlier than 13 weeks gestation, and especially those of the fundus, often resolve without intervention; but some perforations, especially those which encounter arteries or which involve non-sterile instruments, can be life-threatening.[12]

---

11 Edelman, D. and Berger, G. (1981) In: Hodgson, J. Abortion and sterilization: medical and social aspects New York: Grune and Stratton p.217 archive.org/details/abortionsterilizoooounse
12 Kaali, S.G., Szigetvari, I.A., & Bartfai, G.S. (1989). The Frequency and Management of uterine perforations during first trimester abortions. American Journal of Obstetrics & Gynecology, 161(2), 406-8

Air introduced into the uterus might lead to fatal perforations or emboli. The one-way valve of the Del-Em is perhaps one of its most important features. Make sure the Del-Em is functioning correctly.

Incomplete abortion, a failure to remove all products of conception, can lead to hemorrhaging, infection, and/or continued pregnancy.

Conflict surrounding unwanted pregnancy and its familial and state politics can be extremely disturbing to emotional health. Lability, anxiety, depression, and suicidality can result, and so emotional support and prolonged follow-up is strongly urged.

Jailtime, fines, and public scorn are a possibility for anyone practicing menstrual extraction.

The Anatomy of Self-Help

Self-help groups typically encourage a step-wise learning process where participants advance their skills in order to engage safely in menstrual extractions. Attendees absorb group culture and knowledge at meetings, seminar-like clinics, and during actual menstrual extractions. They learn to readily identify pelvic anatomy. They perform cervical self-exams and then progress to pelvic exams and uterine palpation with partners. They memorize the menstrual extraction process, and are able to identify risks, contraindications, possible complications that might arise, and readily formulate plans to handle all scenarios. Moving forward, participants would allow the group to perform a menstrual extraction on themselves, and participate in others' menstrual extractions.

This may seem radical, *and it is radical*—in a good way! After jumping hurdles of reservation, shame, and shyness, participants unlock new worlds of freedom, knowledge, ability, and self-acceptance. They're less detached from and helpless about their physical bodies, and they're fully initiated into a trustworthy support group akin to a second family. They have someone to call *if...*

I like this style of learning. One thing I've learned over the years is that I'm able to provide much more thoughtful, compassionate care to patients when I myself have experienced what they are going through. Before we stick things in other people, it's best we poke ourselves first—not just for practice and to learn what might feel better, but to build empathy. I understand it might seem "weird" to a lot of people to so-to-speak communalize anatomy lessons and reproductive care, but it really does pay off to see firsthand just how much we all have in common, and take back control over our bodies.

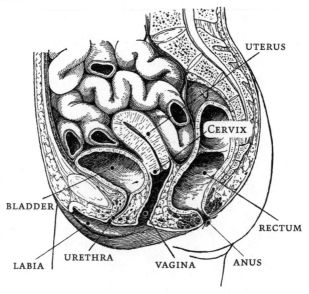

For self-help purposes, it's crucial to have an understanding of female anatomy such that we are able to find the vaginal opening, the cervix, and the cervical opening (os). Furthermore, practicing with our eyes, hands, and speculums, we will begin to appreciate differences in anatomy such as uterine size or position, or clues such as the color of the cervix or texture of cervical mucus, which provide valuable information or even warnings prior to performing menstrual extraction. As we practice we become more curious, outgoing, and more able to not only speak with others about what's been learned, but to find consensual partners (if not just yourself) for more hands-on practice. Many people will be surprised to learn that with the right tool, the cervix is as accessible as that little dangly uvula thing in the back of our throats.

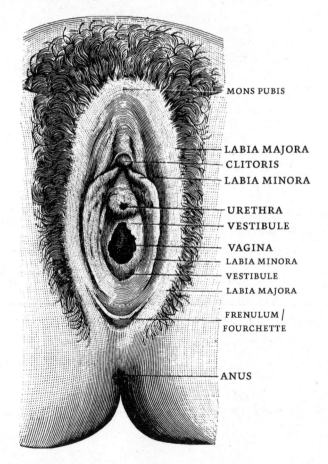

MONS PUBIS

LABIA MAJORA
CLITORIS
LABIA MINORA

URETHRA
VESTIBULE

VAGINA
LABIA MINORA
VESTIBULE
LABIA MAJORA

FRENULUM /
FOURCHETTE

ANUS

If you have a cervix, you can learn how to do a cervical exam on yourself. If you have a partner with a cervix, you can ask permission to do a cervical exam and maybe also practice a bimanual (two hand) exam to palpate (locate and feel) pelvic organs. A bimanual exam can be used to locate and describe uterine size and position. This skill later becomes crucial in deciding whether or not to perform a menstrual extraction at all.

Let's start by reviewing where the vaginal opening is found. Looking at the preceding illustration, be aware it was created by a medical illustrator referencing a pinned cadaver, not a live model. Just like a butterfly does not rest with its wings wide open without being pinned, the outer and inner labia, and the vagina do not naturally splay and gape open. If it's *your* vagina you're going to look at, you can squat over a mirror and pull back your labia to find the opening; it's about halfway between your clitoris ("love button") and your anus ("butthole"). Also find the urethra, which is just above / in front of the vagina, and sometimes even *slightly* inside the vagina. You'll want to be able to locate both, because down the road you don't want to be trying to insert a finger or speculum in a urethra. Ouch!

If you can't look now or haven't seen many vulvas, peep the late great Betty Dodson's vagina illustrations in "Sex for One," or search "Great Wall of Vagina" on the Internet. You will see there is a wide and wonderful variety in shapes and sizes – no two vulvas are alike. The goal is to have a working knowledge of what is what anatomically, no matter whose vulva you are looking at.

Manual Cervical Exam

The manual (using a hand) cervical exam is the simple act of inserting one or two fingers into the vagina to palpate the vaginal walls and cervix, and, in more complex exams, to rule out problems with the vaginal wall or structures like muscles and glands that surround it. Grow comfortable with the following steps because other self-help skills build on them, and they will be breezed over later.

You and/or your exam partner might feel nervous about manual exams. It's right to be careful with one another and move slowly, but in order to learn skills required for confident and safe menstrual extractions, hands-on practice is necessary. For various totally valid reasons, some people have reservations about looking at a crotch or inside a vagina, or having theirs seen. It gets easier each time you look or are looked at, especially as you see how similar we all are "down there."

People insert tampons, menstrual cups, dildos, probes, penises, pessaries, and other things in vaginas, but it takes curiosity and a shedding of accumulated fear and shame to become more familiar using fingers and eyeballs. Maybe look that shame right in the eye; it's holding you back from understanding and guarding a vital part of our bodies. Our vaginas deserve attention, too!

Still struggling with it? It really helps to take some time to make an inventory of hangups, and work through them as gently as possible with a close friend or counselor. Sometimes it just takes time. Your self help group should work with you so you can view exams repeatedly until you feel comfortable enough to be examined. In cases where a history of vaginal pain, gender dysphoria, genital mutilation, or sexual trauma exists, advanced examination skills and heightened compassion are requisite. This means if you suffer from one of these issues, you deserve extra TLC during examination.

Have the examinee urinate before a pelvic exam. Wash your hands with soap and running water. Gather rubber or nitrile exam gloves if working with a partner, and lubricant. If you are not examining yourself, have the examinee lay on their back on the floor or on a table, and ask them to spread their knees wide (never do it for them). If examining yourself, standing upright is sometimes easiest, especially if you have short arms or padding.

Before the examination, maybe ask something like, "Is there anything I should know about before I take a look?" This opens the door for sharing and might head off any surprises later. As you proceed with an exam, explain what you plan to do before you do it, and assure the examinee is comfortable and consenting throughout. "I'm looking at your skin texture and color, seems normal. Is it OK to touch your vulva now? I'm feeling for... etc. Especially if you are familiar with normal, healthy anatomy, reassure the examinee that what you are seeing is normal. With an attitude of curiosity, break any surprising findings after the exam, when the examinee is clothed again.

Apply a coin-sized spot of lube to the forefinger and middle fingers of your dominant hand. Hold your hand palm facing up and tuck the fingers you won't be using tight into your palm. You may need to gently separate the labia majora a bit to expose the introitus (vaginal opening); you can do this with a thumb and forefinger in a spreading motion. "Touching, you will feel pressure, let me know if anything hurts." Avoid speaking words which could have sexual connotation. Be conscientious of any tender spots or positions, which might become obvious by wincing, recoiling, and/or vocalizations such as "ow!"

The vaginal walls will feel similar to the inside of your cheek and lips. The cervix, shaped a little like a one-inch half donut round, should be the only feature that pops out at you, both soft and firm like pursed lips, at the far end of the vagina. If you cannot feel the cervix, bearing down (as if to poop) might help drop it into reach. You can trace its circumference with your finger, and find the os (opening) in its center. This incredible bundle of muscle is capable of stretching open to pass a baby's head and shoulders and selectively allows menstrual blood and semen to pass, yet is otherwise a protective gatekeeper to the uterus.

Take note of the size and shape of the cervix, and the shape of the cervical opening. Can you tell from the size and shape whether a person might have had a pregnancy before? Also observe its color, any texture, and the appearance of mucus on the cervix. Is it clear? Milky? Pink or brown-tinged? Bloody? Where is the examinee in their menstrual cycle (if they are still menstruating)?

If you have permission and a long cotton-tip applicator (Q-tip), you can check out the viscosity of the mucus. Is it milky? Is it clear? Is it stretchy and watery like egg white? Gummy and dry? Maybe ask the examinee what mucus has been like the past couple days. If you're really curious, smell it. You might be surprised to learn most cervical mucus barely has a scent.

It can get really interesting and ultimately useful to track these observations with different women at different points in their cycle, and hopefully pregnant women, too. You can learn how the cervix and mucus change appearance over the month and during pregnancy. Eventually, and with some study on the side, you will be able to add cervical assessment to your gestation calculation.

One last thing: does the examinee wish to see their own cervix? You can help them with a hand mirror, or with their consent, take a picture for them with their phone camera.

Move confidently and pay attention to what you are perceiving so you can move efficiently forward with your exam. A quick exam is almost always a more comfortable experience. That said, don't rush. Involve the examinee in any discussion and reassure them about the "within-normal" parts of the exam. Provide a tissue or wet wipe as a courtesy, and give thanks to the examinee for volunteering. You're learning so you can help others!

Note: Be conscious how, as you grow more and more accustomed to performing these intimate exams, you become more comfortable doing them. One trap is becoming so comfortable that you cycle people through like sheep, neglecting their uniqueness and discomfort. Try to approach each person afresh, and remember nobody really enjoys getting a pelvic exam.

The Speculum

Simply put, speculums are used to hold body holes open. There are speculums for noses and buttholes, but the vaginal speculum is probably best known. Vaginal speculums are fairly easy to obtain and I gotta say, great to have on hand. My brother found mine (a vintage stainless steel relic) at a dump, clean and in its original bag. Speculums can be bought cheap online. Get one "free" at your next annual exam by showing your provider a gallon-size Ziploc and requesting they place your used plastic speculum inside when finished. Heck, some sex shops even sell speculums (not exactly a big detour given the devices' *interesting*, lurid history)![13]

Speculums typically come in four sizes: extra small through large, medium being most common. Another way to think of the small, medium, and large sizes are: narrow, medium, and long. The small size is sometimes used for older people and teenagers. The large size is occasionally helpful for those who have birthed children, or overweight or obese people. That said, there is no correlation between body size and vagina size. It's just that sometimes there is more tissue to hold aside in order to create a view of the cervix, and wider bills help with that. Use whatever size works to get a view of that cervix.

Speculums are either plastic or metal, but they are otherwise mostly the same shape these days. Except for some really cool new designs made by people with vaginas for people with vaginas... but those might be difficult to get your hands on. A lot of people prefer

13 Eveleth, R. (Nov 17 2014) "Why No One Can Design a Better Speculum" *The Atlantic* web.archive.org/web/20220323195842/ TheAtlantic.com/health/archive/2014/11/why-no-one-can-design-a-better-speculum/382534/

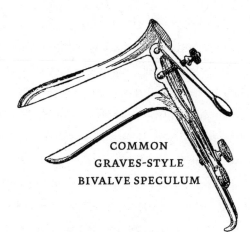

COMMON
GRAVES-STYLE
BIVALVE SPECULUM

plastic speculums if only because they are warm where stainless steel is cold. Then again, a lot of people hate the ratcheting sound plastic speculums make. It's a bit early to become a speculum connoisseur, but I hope you eventually find your favorite.

Even though plastic speculums are marketed as disposable, they can be washed and reused until they crack. Wash your speculum, plastic or metal, with soap and water soon after use, and rinse well.

Speculums often have two adjustments: one to increase the viewing/tunnel height, and another which separates the bill tips (avoid calling them blades) in a jaw-opening fashion. A speculum can be inserted with the handle facing up or down per your preference. Start with bills fully closed and at a 45° angle from horizontal. Tip into a final handle-up or handle-down position while inserting. Once inserted, many users will adjust the viewing height first, and if the cervix doesn't pop into view, they might pull the speculum out slightly in case a bill is over the cervix. If they feel vaginal wall tissue is in the way, they might increase the jaw angle with the second adjuster and find the cervix revealed. With a see-through plastic speculum, you can sometimes see the cervix through a bill and know where to adjust. So long as the cervix isn't pinned between the bills, it's friendlier to collapse the speculum slightly before making adjustments, then expand it again when in place.

Speculum adjusters can be awkward to operate, so I recommend practicing on a pair of socks before practicing on a vagina. A pair of socks? Yes, a pair of tight, mid-length socks! Put one sock over your hand and arm, then pull another sock up on top of the first. Now fold both socks down about ⅓ of the way back toward your hand, and then fold again, at which point a closed-ended sock tube will probably pop off your hand, hopefully 4-6 inches long. Hold the tube with your non-dominant hand somewhat firmly, because in fact vaginal wall muscles will resist the prying speculum. If you're dexterous you can simulate a cervix at the closed end with a fingertip.

Run your sock "vagina" through a mock exam. Get your headlamp or flashlight and maybe even lubricate the speculum bills. Vocally walk the sock through what it might feel next. "This might feel cold." When opening the speculum, you can say, "pressure."

Always spread the bills and clear the cervix first before collapsing the bills to move or remove the speculum. Also avoid pinching the sides of the vaginal wall while you collapse the speculum to remove it or change its position. Release the adjusters gradually. Sometimes rotating the speculum slightly back and forth while releasing and closing helps prevent pinching. While it's still just a sock you're examining, build some speculum finesse and confidence!

Wait, do you feel like this sock has a lot of sock in the way of your view and you maybe need a bigger speculum to hold back the sock? If you don't have a larger speculum, there's a fun new trend that might help: placing a condom on the speculum, cutting off its tip, and then inserting the speculum with a tip-less condom.[14]

14 Freeman, L. (April 2018) Canada Family Physician Condom use to aid cervical visualization during speculum examination

The condom sheath prevents the vaginal walls from collapsing into view, and can also help with comfort. Put that in your toolbox.

Note: inserting a speculum into oneself is often easier than letting someone else do it. That's great news for self-exams, but also a courtesy you can maybe offer when participating in self-help groups.

Cervical Self-Exam

If you're feeling adventurous and open to finding your own cervix, fetch a hand mirror (or any moveable wall mirror), a headlamp / flashlight / gooseneck lamp, a vaginal speculum, and a little lubricant.

Since I got my landfill-bound speculum about 25 years ago, I've done a lot of quick cervical self-exams. In my mind, these self-exams are similar to taking a close look at my teeth and gums. I do it because I want to catch anything weird, you know . . . before it turns into a root canal.

I'll do a self-exam any day when I'm not menstruating heavily. That just gets messy. But if you're curious, I say go for it.

---

ncbi.nlm.nih.gov/pmc/articles/PMC5897075/

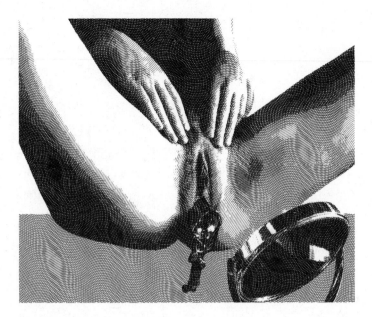

I find self-exam is easiest to do in a hallway, with the mirror propped against one side wall, and myself sitting propped against a pillow on the other side wall. Find what will work for you. Strip from the waist down, sit down on a thick pillow or pile of books, spread your knees wide, and take a second to appreciate the anatomy between your legs. Are you aware and appreciative of how normal, beautiful and incredibly powerful it is? I hope so! Make sure to take note of what you see so you can compare it to next time, and report any questions or concerns to your health care provider... and self-help group.

Squirt your lube of choice (it doesn't have to be sterile for this) on a paper towel and dip the bills of your speculum into the lube a bit, or spread a little directly onto the speculum. Some people will dab some lube directly at the introitus instead, some people will do both. Some people are lucky enough to not need lube, or only use water. Keep it comfortable.

Separate your labia if your vaginal opening doesn't come into view, then insert the speculum. Since you are human and not a sock, you'll want to angle the speculum slightly towards the small of the back while inserting, and put any pressure down towards the bum while moving it because anterior (forward) structures like the urethra are more delicate and irritable. When doing this exam on someone else, it is a kind gesture to put your two first fingers just in front of (anterior to) the fourchette, pull slightly down (posteriorly) towards the anus, and slide the lubricated speculum over your fingertips.

If all you have is a flashlight, it can be placed on a folded towel in front of you and aimed directly into your vagina or its reflection. If you wear a headlamp, shine its light into the mirror.

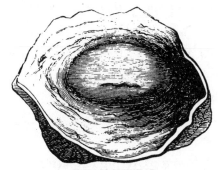

VIEW OF CERVIX AT
THE END OF VAGINA

Open the speculum and center the cervix in view at its end. If you're so lucky as to find your cervix on your first try, great! But it isn't always that easy. It might help to feel inside your vagina with your finger to locate your cervix, then re-aim the speculum. Don't give up. It might take some wiggling, speculum re-positioning, and practice, but it's worth it. Once you get there, admire yourself—this is some way cool stuff you're doing and seeing! Over the years a cervix will change, and without taking a look ourselves, we'd miss out. You now have the power to watch for normal changes, as well as untoward changes like pus, warts, polyps or surface weirdness that might indicate cancer.

> *"We must get rid of that attitude of dependency on doctors for our healthcare and realize that it is our body. If we don't learn about our own bodies, somebody else is going to be in charge of what happens to us. It's just that simple."*
>
> ~Carol Downer[15]

Bimanual Exam for Uterine Palpation

An anatomy-based skill that expands with practice is uterine size estimation by palpation. Palpation means feeling of inner body structures like the uterus by prodding with fingers. It's a dying skill in the age of ultrasound and medical imaging, but in the absence of that technology, it's a very valuable skill. If you've been to the doctor's, you've probably had your belly palpated. They might have been feeling around for a growth, maybe an enlarged liver, or just pressing around to see if you experienced discomfort anywhere.

Obviously a bimanual pelvic exam is quite a bit different from just having a belly prodded, since it involves a gloved hand, lubricant, and vaginal penetration. It is also quite difficult to do on yourself, so find a partner. Continue gently and with consent.

15 Baker, C.N. *Abortion How-To: The Ms. Q&A on Menstrual Extraction With Carol Downer* Ms. Magazine July 14 2022

Have your partner pee first, and get into a comfortable reclined position. It's wise to *begin* by palpating the person's lower belly to check for tenderness, bloating, masses, hernias, wounds or scars, or tenderness.

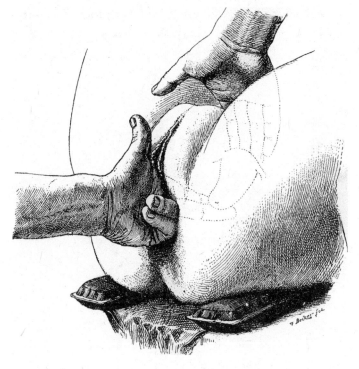

After palpating their belly, have them spread their knees wide, so that you will be able to position yourself between their legs. In the image above, the examiner has fingers of their stronger/dominant hand externally on the top (fundus) of the uterus, and fingers of non-dominant (left) hand behind the cervix at the end of the vagina. There are physical reasons to use the left hand inside the vagina during a bimanual exam,[16] but ultimately this might come down to what you are comfortable with. In the image, the examiner pushes the uterus up towards the outside hand for palpation. Most of the time, the uterus will feel firm and moveable.

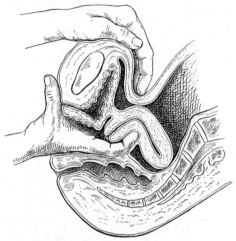

RETROFLEXED UTERUS

As a beginner, or even as an estimation-by-palpation hotshot, it's helpful to understand that this is a complicated "art." Palpating uterine size accurately can be made difficult by factors like obesity, uterine fibroids,

16 Long WN. Pelvic Examination. In: Walker HK, Hall WD, Hurst JW, editors. Clinical Methods: The History, Physical, and Laboratory Examinations. 3rd edition. Boston: Butterworths; 1990. Chapter 177.

or a history of several pregnancies. More commonly the uterus is draped forward over the urinary bladder (anteverted or anteflexed) and can be felt between the low belly and fingers inside the vagina. Sometimes you won't be able to palpate the uterus easily at all due to it being retroverted (tilted) or retroflexed (flexed) back toward the rectum. In that case, fingers inside the vagina are too far forward to catch the uterus' height between themselves and fingers of the opposite hand. A retroverted or retroflexed uterus is sometimes concomitant with a cervical os that aims forward (anteriorly) rather than backward.

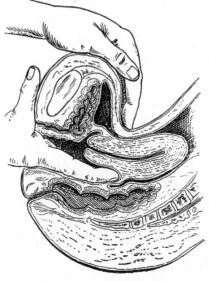

RETROVERTED UTERUS

Until 6 weeks' gestation or so, changes in the uterus won't really be palpable. But at six weeks, the uterus will be a couple centimeters larger than usual, and will grow a centimeter each week thereafter. Do enough bimanual exams on non-pregnant volunteers, and you will have a good basis for estimating uterine growth on pregnant ones. If you can find pregnant volunteers for estimation practice, even better. If, using one hand to palpate the low belly just above the pubic bone, you can easily feel a rounded, firm uterus poking up and out below thin layers of skin and fat and muscle, it's likely pregnancy is beyond first term (>12 weeks)… and self-help menstrual extraction is definitely not appropriate.

This skill truly depends on attuned practice, and safe ME depends on this skill. After a lot of bimanual exam experience, your fingers will relay messages about uterine size and quality to your brain, which can fairly accurately gauge gestation, if it exists. Palpation is also important to rule out pelvic pain or masses, which would contraindicate ME, and warrant a doctor's visit.

The "Del-Em" Menstrual Extraction Kit

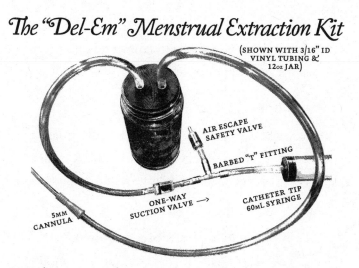

(SHOWN WITH 3/16" ID VINYL TUBING & 12oz JAR)

AIR ESCAPE SAFETY VALVE

BARBED "T" FITTING

ONE-WAY SUCTION VALVE →

CATHETER TIP 60mL SYRINGE

5MM CANNULA

A Del-Em is such a simple, small, DIY tool, but it represents a recapturing of body rights which have been at times withheld and at other times presented as shameful, expensive, dangerous and unapproachable. It's a mascot of reproductive rights!

We recommend you build one and keep it on hand, because building one rapidly on demand could be tough. Some parts may take longer to find, or might cost more than you can budget this month. The double/dual air check valve pictured on the cover is very difficult to find these days, so I'll give instructions for how to build a Del-Em with two simple and cheap air check valves instead.

There are several ways to assemble a Del-Em. Have fun and get creative with connectors found at the hardware store.

You'll need:

- A round clear glass jar, at least 6 oz but it doesn't need to be any bigger than 12 ounces. Taller than it is wide. 8oz regular mouth canning jars work great.

At your local hardware store, or online:

- A rubber cork to fit the glass jar top snugly, without falling in, or popping out when bumped. Some corks will come with two holes pre-drilled. Larger sizes aren't always stocked at hardware stores. Google: "rubber stopper" and look for one the right size, with two holes. Size #13 (58-68mm) will fit a regular mouth canning jar; size #12 (54-64mm) is another regular mouth-sized option if you can't find #13.

- 4 feet of 3/16" ID (internal diameter) clear vacuum tubing in vinyl or silicone, usually sold by the foot. Vacuum tubing has more rigid walls so that it does not collapse under vacuum pressure.

- Barbed Y- or T-shape fitting with ¼" barb, brass or plastic, to accept vacuum tubing

- Barbed coupler fitting with ¼" barb, brass or plastic, to attach cannula to tubing (optional)

At your local pet (aquarium) store, or online:

- Two air "check" valves which will accept your vacuum tubing on both ends, usually ¼". Air enters and exits in only one direction. These are cheap and can be easily found at Amazon and eBay. Read the reviews before buying; some of these valves *whistle loudly.*

Online, at your local medical supply store:

- A 50 or 60 milliliter needleless syringe, catheter (cone) tip. A luer-lock tip syringe can also work.

Through a nurse/doctor ally:

- Several Karman cannulas, in a 4-8 millimeter diameter range[17]

---

17 Before Karman had his cannulas manufactured, he created his by cutting notches with a razor blade in easily obtained medical suction and drain tubing. He never patented the style. As of this writing, only people with a medical license can obtain Karman cannulas in the United States. Building a strong self-help network in your area improves chances one amongst your group has access to medical supply and/or has stockpiled supplies.

How to Assemble Your Del-Em

1. If your rubber cork doesn't already have holes, drill two holes in it, spaced equally apart and away from the edges of the cork. The holes should be smaller in diameter than your vacuum tubing, but allow the tubing to pass through with some force and a little bit of lubrication (use soap suds, not vaseline or silicone). A nice alternative is to cut two 2" pieces of more rigid tubing to push through the cork, like the type of tubing inside spray and soap squirt bottles. It should be a smaller diameter than your tubing, so you can connect your vacuum tubing.

MedGyn sells a Karman cannula, product # 022004K - 022012K. They're not cheap and must be ordered by your medically-licensed ally. MedGyn also offers various other related supplies (such as cervical dilators and tenaculum) that could make ME easier, but which medicalize it. (medgyn.com)

IPAS Easygrip® cannulas are designed to work with IPAS MVA kits, but can be used with a Del-Em.

In the near future, someone with access to a 3D printing modeler could potentially model a set of Karman cannulas. Autoclavable (read: sterilizable) 3D print materials are becoming more available, and with smoothing, I'm hopeful that someday getting a set of Karman cannulas could be as simple as having them 3D printed.

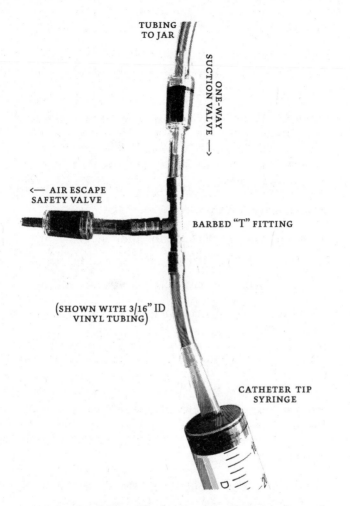

TUBING
TO JAR

ONE-WAY
SUCTION VALVE —>

<— AIR ESCAPE
SAFETY VALVE

BARBED "T" FITTING

(SHOWN WITH 3/16" ID
VINYL TUBING)

CATHETER TIP
SYRINGE

2. Cut a 2" length of vacuum tubing and attach
one end to the syringe tip and the other end
to a barbed Y or T fitting. Cut two more 2"
pieces of tubing and attach both to the open Y

fitting ends. If your tubing at any point seems a tiny bit too small to go onto a fitting, you can heat and soften the end *briefly* with flame from a lighter or match, wet the fitting and press in. Connect a one-way valve to each end, one facing in one direction and one facing the other. The valve that allows air into the syringe will be connected to tubing in step 4. The other valve will allow air out.

3. Cut the remaining vacuum tubing nearly in half, with one end a few inches longer than the other. (It's nice to have a longer cannula end.)

4. With one half of the tubing, attach an end to the valve and insert the other end through the rubber cork and into the jar, about ½"

5. With the other half of the tubing, insert one end through the open hole in the rubber cork and into the jar, about ½" or longer if you have a deep jar.

6. Test your valve setup. If you've put the valve on in the correct orientation, you should be able to fill the syringe with air, but when you push the air out of the syringe it should vent to the surrounding air, *not* out the cannula end.

7. Cannula will attach to the tubing from step 5. Do not attach a cannula until you are ready to use the Del-Em, unless you are willing to sacrifice a cannula for testing or display. Cannulas are not guaranteed sterile unless fresh out of the package. Depending on the cannula, it might mate perfectly with your vacuum tubing. If not, you might have to use intermediate tubing to size up or down. Alternatively you can pick up a small plastic or brass barbed hose fitting at the hardware store to allow fitting various size cannulas.

Fill a glass of water and take your Del-Em for a spin by placing the cannula end of hosing into the glass and pulling suction with your syringe. The jar should begin to fill. When you push your syringe plunger, air should exit the bypass valve, and never create bubbles in the glass of water.

All good? Now place your Del-Em on your mantle… and invite close friends over. *What does it mean to you?,* they'll probably ask. And you'll probably find out what it means to them.

How to Clean and Maintain Your Del-Em

You might not be using your Del-Em frequently, and rubber and plastic degrade over time, so I recommend purchasing new tubing, valves, syringes and cannulas for each use. The only part of the Del-Em which needs to be sterile is the cannula. The rest of it can be "clean enough," but if it's been used you'll want to sanitize it.

Rinse jar, cork and cannula tubing and wash in soapy water. Then the jar and rubber cork can be pressure cooked (at 15psi) for ten minutes, or alternatively, soaked in a 1:10 bleach:water solution for 30 minutes (bleach will eventually break down the cork). Pressure cooking will melt your tubing and cannula.

Test your setup for vacuum and correct pressure direction before each use.

Keep It Clean

Practice "No Touch" on a Papaya

Some self-help and other advocacy groups have great fun using papayas as mock uteruses. Young, green papayas certainly have an uncanny similarity to the human uterus, especially on the stem end, which resembles a cervix when the stem is cored.

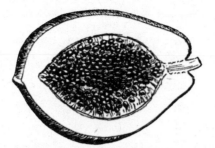

The curious can attempt to pass a cannula into the papaya using "No Touch" technique (e.g. aseptic technique). No Touch is successful if a fruity cervix has been cannulated without touching the cannula tip to anything else but the cervix (and the seeds inside the fruit).

Wipe and and prepare the cervix with a swirly swabbing of antiseptic such as iodine. Only touching one end of the cannula, attempt cannulation. If the cannula touches a table, a thigh, or vagina walls, for example, pretend to replace it with a fresh sterile cannula. Why replace? Because inserting a contaminated cannula into the uterus can increase risk of infection.

Think it sounds easy? Make this more challenging by duct taping a toilet paper roll to the stem end, and get the cannula inserted without touching cardboard!

Unfortunately I've witnessed many professionals botch aseptic technique and have no doubt some of those mistakes caused infections. I urge everyone to carefully study aseptic technique before upgrading from the papaya to a human. I also recommend eating the papaya with some lime squeezed over it—yummy!

Sterile Field Practice

Let's take the idea of aseptic technique beyond papaya practice and imagine creating and using a sterile field. A sterile field is a surface where only sterile items such as instruments and dressings are placed. "Sterile" or "sterilized" means **all** germs on an item have been killed by high heat, such as with steam in an autoclave, or perhaps by using modern low-heat and/or low-moisture methods. Very thin crusts of dirt can be sterilized (because the germs in dirt can be killed) but once something which was once sterile touches dirt or something dirty, it's no longer sterile. If there's so much as a *suspicion* it's no longer sterile, best to treat it like it's probably dirty.

I hate to be a spoilsport, but boiling an item in water on the stove isn't going to truly kill *all* the germs on it. On the other hand, the "poor man's autoclave," a pressure cooker, reaches a temperature at 15psi high enough to kill *most* germs after 15 minutes... and possibly melt the object you're trying to sterilize. While I found it fascinating to learn how the Janes of Chicago sanitized their equipment, I'm not sure I would allow that except in desperate situations.

Starting any procedures with a sterile field is super handy, if only because it sits there, proudly reminding you of "clean" vs. "dirty," and inspires others' confidence in you. Up your game! Sterile towel drapes are cheap and easy to find. An often-cheaper upgrade is the "catheter insertion kit," which doesn't include a catheter but conveniently packages sterile gloves, a drape, and lube.

At the beginning of a procedure, the sterile field is created by laying a sterile drape on a side table, or perhaps covering a cookie sheet which will be kept within reach. Touch only the outer ½-1" of the drape in order to spread it, and then consider that outer perimeter "dirty." Sterile items can be placed inside this perimeter. For example, you could spill out your giant cotton-tipped applicators onto the sterile field. Peel open the sterile item packaging (the packaging has split ends and is designed to cleanly split, front from back) and without touching the item, let it fall onto the field. You can touch the packaging, but don't touch what's inside. Got it?

OK, so now you have some cotton-tipped applicators laying on a sterile field; everything inside the field is still sterile, untouched. You could pour iodine (preferably from a fresh bottle or sterile packets) over the applicator tips. Everything on the sterile field is still sterile, right?

Work through procedures step-by-step and visualize where you will put items which need to be set down temporarily. Are they dirty or clean? Often it ends up that your non-dominant hand gets used for touching and moving "dirty" items, and your dominant hand is entrusted with holding the "clean" cannula and making sure it is not contaminated. Having a trash bin nearby can help prevent mistakes.

Visualize what you would do if someone sneezed on your sterile field (masks are on the supply list). What you would do if you accidentally put a "dirty" object on top of sterile items on your sterile field. Level up by having a partner who is familiar with aseptic technique watch your process. They will call out mistakes you might not notice, such as when you unwittingly scratch your itchy nose or push up your glasses... while wearing sterile gloves.

Good aseptic technique is the best way to prevent outside germs being introduced through the cervix into the uterus. Once you have set up a sterile field, it should not sit unused for more than an hour or two; if curious fingers or paws don't get into it first, germs floating in the air will eventually contaminate it.

Menstrual Extraction Step-by-Step

By now you have an understanding of some anatomy and concepts, and have hopefully found or begun building your own self-help network who have also done their reading and research. You will have practiced in your head and then in person, performing ME on fellow non-pregnant members and hopefully having your own ME to opt out of a monthly period. You will have discussed successes and failures with one another, and bonded over common goals. You will have all memorized and be able to work together through the steps of pelvic exams and menstrual extraction. The person having the menstrual extraction (the "extractee") might be skilled enough to lead, in which case, follow that lead... and behold empowerment embodied!

Be aware it's extremely difficult to perform ME safely on yourself, alone. Just imagine being stuck in an awkward reclined position with a speculum in your vagina. That pretty much pins you down. You've only got two hands, say your right hand is your "clean hand," and something you need is out of reach on your right side. Furthermore, remember everything is reversed in the mirror, and you've got to somehow insert a cannula in your own cervix without touching it to anything but your cervix and uterine cavity. You move right and your reflection moves left, and your cannula has brushed the speculum and your thigh. Ugh. Find a helper!

Please understand that this guide is brief. Any book on menstrual extraction, no matter how long, would be incomplete due to the vast possible combinations of conditions, bodies, personalities, and treatment plans. Follow up this reading by poring through the Recommended Reading section, and seek out study buddies and mentors who can reinforce your critical thinking skills and keep you out of trouble.

Gather Supplies

- A Del-Em kit

- A speculum

- Flashlight and/or headlamp and/or gooseneck lamp

- Packaged Iodine swabsticks (at least 4" long) – OR – a bottle of iodine and longer, large headed swabs (like GIANT Q-Tips) – OR – a bottle of iodine, cotton balls, and ring "sponge" forceps or tongs

- Disposable bed pad such as chucks, or something absorptive and maybe waterproof (such as a new kitchen trash bag laid flat with dark-colored towels folded on top) to put on mattress under hips to prevent linen staining

- Sterile towel drape (individually packaged, non-fenestrated)

- 2-3 packets of sterile, medical grade, water-based lubricant

- 2-3 packets of sterile 2x2 or 4x4 gauze (for clearing clots)

- At least 3 pairs of sterile gloves, for when touching cannula

- Non-sterile nitrile/rubber exam gloves

- Face masks

- Fine mesh strainer

- Clear glass deep baking dish

- Tweezers or skewer

- Magnifying glass (optional)

Comfort Items
- Ibuprofen, Aleve, or Aspirin

- Hot water bottle

- Drinking water

- Pillows, sheets, blankets

- Towels, wash cloths, paper towels, tissues

- Maxi pads

Mental Supplies

There may be bumps in the road ahead, but you will brainstorm together and recover wisely, with safety at the forefront. Remember, many doctors, nurses, medical assistants, and lay people have already performed ME, and *so can you*. Preparation is key. Memorize the steps. Run through the scene in your head before you begin. Anticipate surprises and be open to learning from them.

Ask yourself what you might do if someone knocks on the door or the phone rings. What if the power goes out? What if an instrument breaks? What if you suddenly feel woozy or sick to your stomach? What if someone faints? What is the backup plan for if it doesn't work or something goes wrong? Who will you hand care over to, should you not be able to continue?

Prepare the Setting

Make sure everyone eats as they normally would and hydrates well both before and after the procedure. That said, be cautious allowing snacking during the procedure as fainting, and therefore choking, could be a risk. Offer NSAIDs like Advil (Ibuprofen), Aleve (Naproxen), or Aspirin at least 30 minutes before starting if desired. NSAIDS usually help relieve cramping pain, but Tylenol will not.[18]

Maybe there are soothing changes of setting that could be made, such as closing blinds, adjusting the lighting, locking doors, turning off phones, turning on favorite music at low volume, burning incense, etc. Offer to make tea, and while you're boiling water, fill a rubber hot water bottle (not too hot!) to soothe cramping and ease pain.

Does the extractee consent for everyone who is present to be present and to view? Ask that all observe the extractee's wishes. Make sure everyone is introduced, and maybe wear name tags to make calling out easier in case new friends are present. If anyone present is prone to fainting on the sight of blood, have them chug 16-20 ounces of juice or electrolyte drink before starting, and seat them in a chair.

---

18 ipas.org/clinical-update/english/pain-management/pain-management-for-vacuum-aspiration/

Interview

If you have not already, proceed with an interview to become familiar with the extractee's health history. You will want to know about:

- Age

- Number of pregnancies and births

- Date of last normal menstrual period

- Date of conception (if known and if applicable)

- All drugs used daily or recently. Prescription and non-prescription drugs, herbs, vitamins, etc.

- Alcohol, marijuana, and other illicit drug use, as well as caffeine and tobacco use

- Allergies or adverse reactions to drugs, foods, and other substances

- Medical history, especially endocrine, cardiac, and/or bleeding disorders

- Surgical history, especially pelvic or abdominal surgery

- Recent pelvic exam, pap smear and/or STD test results, if available. Is there a history of warts, cervical polyps, endometriosis, cesarean births, scarring, retroverted uterus, heavy bleeding, pain?

- How are they feeling? What is their attitude at the moment? What are their goals for the procedure and goals for how they want to feel after the procedure? Do they have fears? Are they prone to anxiety attacks? What can calm them? Any special requests?

- Confirm everyone's contact information. Will you be able to reach them for follow-up?

This is a lot of information. Keep organized by taking notes, and refer to them periodically. I suggest you do not include identifying information in your notes. Keep the notes in a safe, private place until you have confirmed the extractee is doing well a few weeks later. Notes can reassure you if questions come up later, and help you to learn.

During the interview, evidence may come to light which should bring pause. Are there hints that there may be difficulty or risk in cervical cannulation, such as the extractee being young and nulliparous (never having given birth)? Known anteflexed or retroflexed uterus? Are there clues there may be extraordinary anxiety or pain during the procedure, such as the extractee having a history of drug abuse or pro-life religiosity? Could there be a sudden physiologic response to stress of the procedure due to a cardiac or endocrine problem? Is there an abusive or controlling romantic partner or family member who could create drama, and possibly legal issues?

Be alert for any pieces of the puzzle that just don't fit; unfortunately some people might be so desperate for an abortion they will lie about their gestation and medical history. Any concerns should be run through carefully, weighing risk against the team's skill, capability and keeping in mind that surprises might arise. The word-of-mouth, family/friends network nature of self help groups tends to keep these discussions honest, but don't get so comfortable that you miss red flags. It is best to not perform ME when your gut, or your self-help group, is telling you something is "off."

In the interview, which is perhaps more wisely done earlier by phone call, you will have determined a gestational age. It's awesome when someone can tell you the exact moment they last bled or that they conceived, but if not, do some careful counting on the calendar. Your final cannula size selection depends on the gestational age, with a fairly straight across weeks:millimeters ratio, plus or minus one millimeter. 5 weeks: 4-6mm. 6 weeks: 5-7mm, etc. If you don't have the correct size sterile cannula to match the gestational age, or uterine palpation belies gestation weeks beyond the estimated gestational age, you should stop here.

After the interview, encourage the extractee into a comfortable, sustainable position which will allow a pelvic exam and the insertion of a speculum and cannulas. There will be times you need them to hold still, and other times you can offer them to shift their weight and get comfortable again. Offer a blanket or sheet to drape over belly and knees, providing a degree of warmth and/or privacy. At a point when they seem calm, you might take a pulse (count heartbeats for 30 seconds and multiply by 2 to get beats per minute) to establish a baseline heart rate. Are they pale? Pink? Is their skin warm? Do they complain of feeling cold? If there is a lot of bruising, could it be possible they have a bleeding disorder, or worse, could there be physical abuse occurring? It's smart to snap a mental picture now, so that if, for example, you are concerned about bleeding later you can decide if they have gotten paler, colder, or their heart rate has shot up. Keep in mind they might just be pale with squeamishness or discomfort and their heart might be racing with anxiety or fear. Use the clues alongside your intuition, and ask questions.

For the next part, you will need your gloves, lubricant and speculum. Maybe postpone setting up your sterile field until after the bimanual exam is complete. Wash your hands, wrists and forearms thoroughly with soap and running water and put on a pair of exam gloves (non-sterile is fine).

Anxiety not only aggravates itself, but also the perception of pain, so do your best to maintain a calm and self-assured tone. Ensure that all participants understand and agree with the plan. Keep the extractee in the loop, sharing information and making eye contact where possible. Every person is different, but most do not like to be left in the dark, especially not with their naked parts hanging out! Respect their feedback and wishes. If they want to stop, just stop.

Begin with a visual exam of the external genitalia, looking for blisters, lesions or sores, or even swollen inguinal (groin) lymph nodes. These might alert you to infection, and a higher risk of passing infection into the uterus. If the visual exam is within normal range, follow with a bimanual exam to assess for any pre-existing pelvic pain, and even more importantly, to gauge uterine size.

If you find evidence of infection or advanced gestational age, report it to the extractee and other participants in a kind but matter-of-fact way and reconsider continuing. If other capable people are present and the extractee consents, you might elicit a second opinion. People are empowered by facts and need them in order to make sane decisions.

Cannula Preparation

Prepare a sterile field. On one corner of the sterile field, swabs or cotton balls can be doused in iodine. On another corner, squeeze out a packet of lube or two. Remember, once your sterile field is set up, it's best to err on the side of having too much supply than too little. Below the lube on one side, spill out one of your smallest size cannula. Leave room for other sizes to be spilled onto the field by your helper *as you need them*. Because new-in-package sterile cannulas aren't easy to come by, you won't want to open them until you are sure you'll be using them. Smaller cannula sizes might not be good for extracting tissue chunks; however, they will help with gradual dilation of the cervix.

Ultimately, it's more up to the extractee how big a cannula will be tolerated, but make good effort to go up to a size in millimeters at least matching gestational age in weeks unless you've already confirmed all gestational tissue is removed with a smaller size.

Bolder practitioners might lay out other instruments on their sterile field, but I will leave that up to you because things really start to get "medical" at that point. Everyone has a preference for how they like to "map" their sterile field or supplies. Personally I put early prep items like iodine on one side, and items I will need throughout the procedure on the other. The prep side becomes the dirty side of my sterile field once prep is finished.

Antiseptic Preparation
Insert a speculum (or allow the examinee to insert a speculum) and isolate their cervix in view. You're probably an expert at this now but one last little trick: if you struggle to find a heavier person's cervix, it sometimes helps to have them bring their knees toward their chest. Make sure you have plenty of light, a good view, and a comfortable position to sit in for yourself. You have two choices here: 1) you can forfeit a corner of your sterile field by taking swabs off it with a non-sterile gloved hand, or 2) you can put on and essentially waste sterile gloves which will only be used for this step. I usually choose to forfeit the corner, and remember to

myself that the iodine corner of the field is no longer clean. (If that's not a confusing irony, I don't know what is.)

Fetch an antiseptic swab, hopefully sopping wet with antiseptic. Insert it into the vagina until it is touching the cervical os, then begin to paint a spiral outward towards yourself. Don't reverse your painty swabbing, and don't overlap by much if at all. Go ahead and swab the speculum along with the vaginal walls as you swirl all the way outside their body. Discard the swab, preferably directly into a trash bin but definitely not on the sterile field. (There's dirty, and then there is dirty dirty! Anything with body fluids on it that cannot be sterilized goes directly in the trash.) Fetch a second swab and repeat, and then finish with a third swab. Iodine has a long history being a safe and effective antiseptic, and you're unlikely to encounter a person allergic to it, but if you do, a non-alcohol antiseptic solution like chlorhexidine can be used instead.

Entering the Sterile "No-Touch" Zone
It is time to put on sterile gloves if you have them. That is a skill in itself and I invite you to watch videos posted online by doctors and nurses showing how to do it correctly. Do you recall any movie or TV where

surgeons are holding their gloved hands up in the air uselessly in front of themselves? Aha! They're doing that to signal that their gloved hands are sterile. It's as much a "stay clear" warming as it is a reminder to the self not to touch anything haphazardly. So be silly and hold up your hands. Go ahead and make a show of how careful you are going to be with the extractee's uterus. Make others aware that your gloved hands are now "clean" (sterile), and invite them to give you a heads up if you touch anything unclean with your dominant hand. Change gloves if that happens. You can touch a sterile cannula with your dominant hand because it's in a sterile glove. Your non-dominant hand will touch "unclean" at some point very soon: a bed sheet, the speculum, the Del-Em, etc., and that's OK. Just focus on keeping a clean dominant hand, and a clean cannula tip.

Grasp the cannula closer to its color-cuffed end with your dominant hand. With your non-dominant hand push the Del-Em tubing into the cannula cuff, assuring a good seal. It might be that the cannula fits inside the Del-Em tubing if the cuff is trimmed off. Plan ahead. If the glove on your non-dominant hand was sterile, it isn't anymore! From the tip where the holes are located, and including at least 5 inches down from that, the cannula must stay clean.

I've nagged that any instrument passing through the cervical os must be sterile, and you are now aware of "best practice." Common knowledge of the early 20th century included thinking the uterus was sterile inside, but we are coming to know that is not necessarily true.[19] Most people have healthy immune systems that slay intruding bad germs. It is up to you to do your best with no-touch technique, but also understand you probably have a little wiggle room and don't panic if you realize you've made no-touch mistakes. Make a note of any mistakes and monitor later for signs of infection such as fever or foul-smelling or discolored discharge.

Cannulating the Cervix

The cervix is a 2-3 centimeter long tube with tight muscular os "gateways" at each end. There is the outer os, which you can see using your speculum, and also an inner os at the border with and inside facing the uterus. The cervix is likely sitting at an angle and possibly has a bit of flex too (sort of like a macaroni noodle, but not quite so bent). You might have judged this angle by palpation and by viewing the cervix, and will inevitably learn more about the angle during cannulation.

19 Baker JM, Chase DM, Herbst-Kralovetz MM. Uterine Microbiota: Residents, Tourists, or Invaders? Frontiers in Immunology 2018 Mar 2;9:208

Cannulating the cervix, especially passing a cannula through the inner os, can cause waves of cramping-type pain. Nausea, sweating, trembling, and/or fainting may occur. Helpers can be of service offering comfort and promoting relaxation: reassuring in soft tones, holding hands, guiding breathing and relaxation, and offering other cozy treats as appropriate. A hot water bottle on the lower tummy is usually helpful. Sometimes a distracting conversation can work wonders; other times quiet is best. Use your intuition but when in doubt, ask.

If you have a puddle of sterile lube on your sterile field, you can dip the cannula tip in it for a light/minimal coating. Ensure you have a great view and good lighting.

Very carefully direct the cannula toward the cervical os as if it's a dartboard bullseye you must not miss. You are trying to keep the cannula from touching anything other than the cervical os. You are also trying to only touch the cannula–and nothing else–with your dominant hand.

Starting with a small diameter cannula can make penetrating the powerful cervix smooth muscle easier.

When inserting a cannula, lubricant helps, as does slightly spinning the cannula while gently pushing forward. If you are struggling, try withdrawing the speculum slightly to reposition the cervix, or place a rolled towel under the extractee's low hips or have them tuck their knees up to improve the angle. Consider pointing the cannula in various *minor* angles other than the angle you suspected. Never force the cannula. Be very gentle. Cramping might really slow down or even prevent cannulation, but the cannula should never be pushed with more force than you might, for example, press a pencil eraser into your eyelid.

Be leery of sudden sharp, piercing pain as it could indicate a perforation of the cervix or uterus. If you've been thorough, gentle, and are using the correct tools correctly, this complication is *very* unlikely. Slow down, stop, and offer everyone a break. Re-group with a plan after having some moments to rest, think, and assess bleeding. Sometimes it happens that the extractee cannot continue due to discomforts, and might even opt to try again another day. If it is still very early in pregnancy (week 4 or 5) it can actually help to try again after a week has passed. The cervix may soften somewhat.

When you succeed in passing through the tight inner os into the uterus, you may feel a sudden slight give, and the cannula will move forward more freely. Don't push any further before taking a note of the measurement mark on the cannula (or estimating the length of cannula outside the cervix if no marks are present). This is your minimum insertion depth; when the cannula isn't inside the uterus at least this far, any suction applied will be directly inside the cervix—unpleasant!

You will meet resistance again, and maybe even get feedback about discomfort, when the tip of the cannula touches the back wall of the uterus. Feedback might even be, "you've hit the back wall." Pull the cannula back about half a centimeter from the point of resistance. Now take a note of the centimeter marking on the cannula at the cervix, and make this your "max" insertion depth. If using a cannula several sizes smaller than your goal size, maybe don't waste time using suction because the cannula will likely clog. Move forward quickly but carefully. Proceed to remove the smaller cannula and insert another size up immediately while the cervix is dilated.

Note: When taking a moment's break for any reason during ME, consider leaving the cannula in place. It's much easier to remove it and dirty it than it is to place it cleanly again.

Managing Del-Em Suction

Ensure the Del-Em is assembled correctly such that air cannot be pumped out the cannula, and make sure the system holds suction (doesn't leak). Have a helper pull suction for you. You can offer the role to the extractee if they are familiar with the menstrual extraction technique. Once the cannula is past its minimum insertion, one or two pulls on a 60 milliliter syringe plunger are often enough to remove all uterine contents. Sometimes it has to be pulled repeatedly. Make sure to keep the jar propped upright in a way such that blood isn't sucked past the cork into the syringe end of the tubing! If enough blood gets past the cork and into the syringe end of the tubing to cause annoyance, disconnect the tubing at the cork/syringe end, pull water through the tubing with the syringe, then empty the syringe into your clear baking dish.

Cannula Motion

Once suction is established, slowly twist the cannula 180° or more back and forth. Avoid trying full rotations, which could cause awkward whipping of the Del-Em tubing and possibly dirty your clean hand. Alternate the twisting with gently moving the cannula slightly in and outward no more than the max or less than the minimum insertion depths. *Be gentle.* When a lot of deep red material comes down the tube very slowly, you may be dealing with a true menstrual period. You might even notice bits of whitish or yellowish tissue in watery fluid as it passes through the plastic tube and into the jar. The material may flow down the tube in batches in a clear fluid in between, ending up in the jar in spurts.

Loss of Suction

If Del-Em tubing comes disconnected or isn't tight or the cannula is accidentally withdrawn while under suction, you can end up with an air leak and loss of suction. Loss of suction is sometimes accompanied by abrupt gurgling in the tubing or small hissing sounds. Double-check all Del-Em connections are snug.

Clogged Cannula

Clogs are unlikely if using Karman cannulas for menstrual extraction. But if nothing is moving through the cannula or tubing despite pulling suction and moving the cannula, and you doubt the uterus is emptied, stop pulling suction. Remove the cannula and see if the holes in the tip are clogged with clots or other tissue. If you have a sterile item good for poking or wiping on your sterile field (e.g. needle, applicator end, or sterile gauze), you can clear the clot. Try to move that tissue into your clear collection dish, since it might be fetal tissue. Maintain "no touch" aseptic technique. If you are clogging, and especially if you failed here with no touch technique, consider continuing with a fresh sterile cannula, one size up.

Completion

You might sense the uterus has emptied based on clues such as being less able to move the cannula due the emptied uterus contracting in size with strong cramping, or the amount of blood in your Del-Em jar. Expect ⅛ to ¼ cup of blood - not very much. At this point the cannula will likely be clear of blood and any tissue. If there is any concern the extractee could be pregnant and further along than originally thought, the cannula can be left in place inside the uterus, and the jar contents quickly (and discreetly, if called for by group conscience) assessed (see below, "Inspecting Uterine Contents"). If you have any reason to believe there has been a pregnancy, then you have more to do: see the end of the next chapter, "Manual Aspiration," for advice on safely completing this procedure.

Ideally, it will become difficult to move the cannula in and out as the uterus shrinks in size and the cervical canal closes up. You may have to pull in order to extract the cannula.

If there is concern about retained products of conception (POC), they could be expelled by cramping within hours, but if not, vigilance and a possible repeat of the procedure might be required. One elegant "feature" of ME is that its main complication, retained POC, is resolved by simply repeating the ME procedure and removing the POC. Symptoms of retained POC are continuing, often foul-smelling spotting and low-grade fever. Rather than repeat, some people switch to medical abortion (abortion pill) to treat an incomplete abortion.

Totally puzzled by post-vacuum procedure symptoms of pregnancy? Keep in mind pregnancy can be ectopic (outside the uterus). With ectopic pregnancy, the uterus will still shed during ME but you won't find POC, and the person will remain pregnant... and in danger of organ rupture. Ectopic pregnancies 100% require a doctor's visit.

Be aware you could have false positive pregnancy tests up to two weeks after an abortion, so be attuned to, and rely on, other bodily signs of pregnancy.

Blood and uterine tissue caught in the jar should be disposed of per the extractee's wishes, keeping in mind it is technically biohazardous waste. Many will allow it to be flushed in the toilet, but some may wish to bring the jar home for a more personal send-off. One more reason to build your Del-Em around a common canning jar that accepts a screw-on lid!

Otherwise, if the cannula is still in place, try elevating the extractee's hips a few inches with a rolled towel, re-attach the Del-Em and see if continued suctioning gives different feedback. Twist the cannula while moving it slightly in and out, but do not push further than you already have and never push harder. It's definitely better to give up for the day than to risk perforating the uterus.

When finally removing the cannula and speculum, reassure the extractee that you are finished and that they have been so strong! You may be truly finished, or you may be finished for the day because of difficulties or uncertainty. Remind them they have your support and continuing care either way.

Do not try to suction away or clean any blood in the vaginal canal or outside the vagina. Provide them with a tissue to wipe away lube and any blood, and support them as they regain their bearings. They will want to wear a maxi pad (not a tampon or cup). Have them take note of their bleeding and other symptoms until they fade completely away, and plan to be in touch with them until that time.

Aftercare

Take loving care of yourself. Take a day or two off work if possible. Eat well, sleep well, and hydrate with water. Allow time to heal.

After a menstrual extraction, spotting may last a day or two.

If a fever or foul vaginal discharge are encountered, consider repeating the ME procedure. If that is refused or does not help resolve symptoms, report to emergency care if you:

- Run a fever over 100.4°F/38°C for over 12 hours, esp. if combined with any of the following:

- Suffer increasing cramping low abdominal pain not relieved by your usual pain control methods

- Have vomiting and diarrhea for over 24 hours

- Pass clots larger than a golf ball

- Have unusual, foul-smelling vaginal discharge

Check in with one another within the first 24 hours, and make contact again a week afterward to make sure everything is still going well.

Ending a Pregnancy

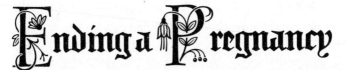

*I*f you've passed the 6 week window for ME, you have other options! Practiced correctly, ME is not an abortion, and can be done without the need to take a pregnancy test, or without pregnancy being your primary concern. But if that pregnancy test is positive and you want out, you still have some (albeit shrinking) options for termination.

Maybe it doesn't need to be said, but I'll say it: there is nothing wrong with choosing an abortion. Some of us don't like babies and don't want to be parents. It's not just a matter of liking babies, though. Child-rearing can be inopportune and difficult. Some choose to not have children because they already have children and cannot financially or physically support more. Some live or work in unsafe conditions. Some might lose their job. Some fear an abusive partner or family members. Some may experience grave physical danger, or even emotional harm, in continuing a pregnancy. Abortion is often chosen in cases of rape and incest. There are many more valid reasons, too. We don't have to explain our reasons to anybody. We can save that energy and use it to take loving care of ourselves during what can be a hard time.

For more ideas about how to protect and take care of yourself before, during and after an abortion, check out The Doula Project's free online zine listed in the Recommended Reading section.

Medication Abortion, or the Abortion Pill

In 2000, the FDA approved an abortion method as simple as taking some pills. Only ten years later the "abortion pill," or "medication abortion" comprised over half of all abortions in the US.[20] It's no wonder these medicines caught on like wildfire in the US; they'd already been used around the world for twenty years. These pills add better affordability and a degree of ease and self-determination to abortion, and avoid surgical procedures.

The prescription medicines mifepristone (a.k.a RU-486) and misoprostol are widely available for medication abortions until 10 weeks gestation, and are sometimes considered for later term abortions or after fetal demise. When taken before 8 weeks gestation, they are effective

---

20 guttmacher.org/article/2022/02/medication-abortion-now-accounts-more-half-all-us-abortions

98% of the time.[21] Doses increase and efficacy drops off the longer pregnancy continues. Bear in mind a medication abortion can prompt an alarming level of cramping and bleeding. It is wise to have guidance so as to know how much is too much.

Mifepristone and misoprostol usually come bundled from the doctor or pharmacy, and are taken within two days of one another as directed by a clinician. It used to be that clinics were required to give the first dose of mifepristone at the clinic, but after repeated challenges this law was reversed in December 2021. This has improved access; however, drastic changes in abortion laws will affect this ruling and many others. Access to medical abortion is in no way guaranteed.

Mifepristone blocks the pregnancy-supporting hormone progesterone, and misoprostol induces cramping and bleeding. In cases where mifepristone is not available, misoprostol can be used alone effectively. Currently, even in places where abortion is illegal, medication abortion is still fairly readily accessible through illegal means. In the US, this often means crossing the border into Mexico to obtain misoprostol,

21 plannedparenthood.org/learn/abortion/the-abortion-pill, pubmed.ncbi.nlm.nih.gov/25592080/

which is also prescribed for gastric ulcers. It should go without saying that illegally obtained medications may not be authentic or pure. The Resources section lists non-profits active in helping people find the real abortion pill.

At the time of writing, the summer of 2022, the legality of medication abortion has gone topsy turvy in the United States. I recommend you obtain these medications now and store them for a time you or a friend might need them in the future, as they may take more time, effort, and money to obtain if anti-choice legislators have their way. Consult the Resources section for advice on medication abortion from the World Health Organization and IPAS.

Abortion Clinics

If we are old enough, have enough money, and are feeling intrepid, we can travel to a clinic where abortion is legal. Clinics licensed to perform abortions generally provide the safest abortion care available. You can use www.abortionfinder.org to locate a provider in the US.

Around the world, some clinics can legally perform elective abortions in clinic up until 22 weeks gestation, but 12 weeks is a more common cutoff.[22] It really depends on where you live, but if you've made up your mind, the sooner you act, the better.

That said, let us first share some warning signs of clinics to avoid, in order to help you get that safe care. Bottom line: be leery of abortion-providing "clinics" who you and your community are not well-acquainted with.

Fake Clinics

Once I went to a "Crisis Pregnancy Center" for a pregnancy test, having no idea that I was in for a strongly biased pro-life lecture, a probing of extremely personal questions, and a piling on of pamphlets and shame, all before even being given the test! It was humiliating. Luckily the test was negative, otherwise their nosey and pushy antics likely would have ramped up several notches.

What was that all about? Turns out, pro-life organizations can pose as fake abortion clinics to intercept people's decision-making. They can lie and trick people in attempts to sway them into choosing to follow through with pregnancies. For example they

---

22 reproductiverights.org/maps/worlds-abortion-laws

may convince someone they have more time to make a decision whether or not to abort, when there actually isn't more time. They often wield shame and guilt as weapons, abusing scripture and/or appeals to morality and family values. Sadly, there may be as many as three times more fake clinics than there are real clinics in the United States, many of them funded by state sale of pro-life license plates... and by federal law they are permitted to deceive you.[23]

If you choose a clinic, peruse the clinic's online reviews for warnings from previous visitors before even calling. If it's still unclear, phone the clinic to ask if they provide abortion services in-office before scheduling. Do they really have a doctor on their premises who performs abortions?

If you still somehow end up at a fake clinic, try not to provide any identifying information, because they might not be trusted with it. If you realize your mistake after arriving, leave without an excuse and do not return. Make sure to fact-check what they have told you, because they will likely have filled your ears with nonsense.

---

23 workers.org/2018/06/37945/

Unacceptable Clinics

When you choose a clinic, remember you have patient rights just as you would at the dentist or doctor's. Legal or illegal, never accept sub-par, unclean, abusive or inhuman treatment! You are still and will always be a gem and worthy of respect, whether you have zero abortions or a hundred abortions. If you encounter any of the following shady practices which might indicate you've landed at an illegal clinic, it's probably best to report them (anonymously) in order to protect other women. Absolutely none of the following should occur in *any* clinic:

- Forcing of contraception method in order to receive abortion

- Verbally or physically abusive staff

- Dirty equipment, dirty or poorly-lit rooms

- Blackmail, extortion, or other threats

- Loss of consciousness without consent

What to Expect at a Legitimate Clinic

Speak with the clinic before arriving and ask if they have any recommendations for self-care before you arrive. The clinic should be able to provide information about:

- Abortion methods available, what they involve, and how long they take

- Ability to accommodate any special needs

- Personal information collected, tests performed, and who information/results are shared with

- Explanation of cramping, pain, bleeding etc. that may be experienced, and which pain medications are available

- Description of normal after-procedure symptoms that might be experienced

- Potential complications and symptoms to watch for, when and how to report

- When sex and other normal activities can be resumed

- Contraception

- Follow-up appointments that might be required

Ask where they recommend you park, and what is the quickest way in and out. Ask if they have trouble with protesters, and if so, if they provide or can recommend escorts. An escort will offer you support getting from your car and in through the front door. No escort? Rally your biggest, best friend or family member who gives the best hugs to accompany you. Do not go alone if you can avoid it, but don't drag along anyone who is shaming you.

I know this can be a tough one, but do not arrive intoxicated.

Waiting in the clinic lobby can be difficult. The atmosphere might feel tense or "off," and conversations with strangers can become awkward—or not! When in doubt, wear noise-canceling headphones and bring a soothing book. Especially if you are alone, play music. Breathe slowly in and out. Remember you are a gem, and worthy of respect.

Keep in mind that similar to the grilling I mentioned in the "fake abortion clinic" section, licensed abortion clinics are generally required by law to ask some pretty pointed, uncomfortable questions about your pregnancy and your decision. If the questions become overwhelming, you can request they ask only the required questions and accept your brief answers when possible. They know that you are probably not having the best day, and hopefully will treat you gently. You will hopefully also understand they are performing often stressful work as best they can. They want to help you, but they've also got many legal hoops to jump through.

You will get through this day and the next. Though you may or may not go through periods of guilt or regret or wondering "what if," your choice at this time is valid and acceptable. Myself and the millions of other women who have made the same choice stand behind you. It is OK.

Outside the Clinic

Although a safe standard in many parts of the world, research shows that people generally prefer to avoid the abortion clinic[24] for various reasons. They find other means to terminate pregnancies, some effective and safe, some not effective or safe.

We do ask that you *do not*:

- Binge on drugs, alcohol or exercise

- Subject your uterus or any other part of yourself to beatings or harm

- Insert anything into your cervix other than correct, proven-safe instruments, with skilled assistance, and under aseptic conditions

---

24 tandfonline.com/doi/pdf/10.1016/S0968-8080(10)36534-7

- Use any caustic chemical or substance in or on yourself

- Use medication outside its recommended dose and purpose

These are harmful, self-disrespectful actions which aren't likely to help bring on your period. Many people die from unsafe abortion attempts every year.

Of the safer, non-clinical means of resuming menstruation, the most common are herbs and menstrual extraction. We will not dive very deeply into herbs here, but please review the reference section for great resources on using them. I'll offer no opinion as to which are the most safe.

Herbs

Herbs are the roots, stems, leaves and flowers of certain non-poisonous *and* poisonous plants, usually used for health benefits or to induce other bodily changes. Some herbs are ubiquitous in our foods, teas, and beauty products, and can be taken in large amounts for long periods without harm. However, the herbs that work to induce menses (emmenagogues) or abortion (abortifacients) are also *poisons*, and must not be taken in quantity or for a length of time. These herbs can be easily found at health food stores, or even foraged and prepared into oils and decoctions and teas at home. The problem is we have no real way of knowing how store-bought herbs were grown and prepared, and how pure and authentic they are. Even if we forage or grow them ourselves, it takes experience and skill to understand how concentrated a "dose" is, and what harm might be done. It's easy to accidentally poison ourselves.

In fits and spurts and too often aligned with trends, scientists explore some herbs' applications, efficacy, safety, and dosing recommendations. Western medical practitioners tend to look down their noses at herbology as an anecdotal pseudo-science. Hand-in-hand with prescribers, the trillion dollar global pharmaceutical market handily sidelines—while borrowing from—sacred herbal knowledge. While some cultures continue to believe in and benefit from natural medicine, few people are able to explain herbology in a way acceptable to the scientific community, much less the FDA.

That doesn't mean herbal medicine isn't valid. Unsurprisingly, emmenagogue and abortifacient herbs contain estrogenic and anti-progesterone compounds similar to synthetics used in birth control pills and medicines like mifepristone. Some grow as "weeds" along roadsides throughout the US. Imagine free birth control for your entire life! People have trusted certain herbs to bring on bleeding for thousands of years. Pills may have an advantage of being consistently formulated and marked with specific dosages, but they are not always as readily available.

There is a narrow window of up to 8-9 weeks gestational age to pursue herbal abortion with emmenagogue and/or abortifacient herbs. The ideal window is within the first two weeks of gestation, when most people are still unaware of being pregnant.

Herbs have helped me bleed (a lot!) several times. I respect their power to both cure *and* kill, and never take them lightly. I urge you to dig deeper into the resources section of *How to Get Your Period* and learn more about herbal abortion. Herbal treatments can powerfully complement a menstrual extraction practice (and vice versa).

Manual Aspiration

There are times when you might be performing menstrual extraction, yet a pregnancy exists. If the extractee is pregnant, you're no longer doing menstrual extraction—this is abortion. Abortion has some very different considerations, legally and medically.

Inspecting Uterine Contents
When performing menstrual extraction, you will not see anything but menstrual blood come out of the Del-Em. If you're curious or concerned or present during an abortion procedure performed after 6 weeks' gestation, you can inspect uterine contents. This is how you do that.

Pour the Del-Em jar contents into a fine mesh strainer and run water over them to rinse away liquid blood. If there is anything left in the strainer after rinsing, move it to a clear glass baking dish, running tap water over the back of the strainer to clear it and to disperse the contents of the dish. With help to hold a flashlight under the baking dish shining upward, inspect the contents.

Products of conception (POC) would include a fetal/gestational sac. This sac surrounds the fetus during pregnancy, and cushions it with fluid. It takes quite a bit of practice to be able to spot the (likely burst and deflated) sac amidst blood clots. Blood clots are generally distinguished by their darker color. If the sac is present, it's not always obvious. It can help to gently stir or poke through the dish with something like tweezers or a skewer, and to look through a magnifying glass. At 6 weeks gestation, the sac might be dime-sized. At 7 weeks gestation, it might be nickel sized, and after that things start to get more obvious. Starting at 9 weeks' gestation, recognizable body parts will be found in the tissue and *must all* be accounted for. Along with the gestational sac you will likely see clotty tissue from the uterine lining (decidua). You may also distinguish some whitish, feathery chorionic villi clouds or tendrils, part of a nourishing connective layer between the fetal sac and uterus.

Manual Aspiration Aftercare

After a manual extraction, bleeding of volume similar or less to a typical period can be expected for up to two weeks and possibly longer. It may only be spotting, and may only last a day or two. There might be a big gush of blood, followed by lighter bleeding. It is also possible that bleeding and cramping are delayed until several days *after* the procedure. Ultimately, the bleeding should taper off.

Uterine (fundal) massage, where the soft part of the abdomen directly above the pubic bone is firmly and deeply massaged, is uncomfortable yet believed by some to encourage uterine cramping and slow bleeding. Fundal massage can be started immediately after ME is complete and for about fifteen seconds a few times a day for a few days afterward if desired.

Until the bleeding has entirely stopped for at least a day, avoid anything penetrating the vagina, such as tampons, silicone menstrual cups, douches, pessaries, penises and sex toys. Baths are OK! If bleeding is just spotty and at least 3 days have passed since the ME, it is OK to resume vaginal penetration. The point here is to let the cervix "gateway" close enough after cannulation and heavy bleeding to prevent germs entering the uterus.

If there is a history of anemia, iron supplementation could be helpful.

If oral contraceptives were being used, resume using a fresh pack, starting with day 1.

You might bleed heavily for a spell. Heavy bleeding soaks a thick maxi pad within an hour. After two hours of heavy bleeding, monitor very closely and get ready to report to emergency care if it continues, especially if accompanied by dizziness, weakness, or fainting. Make it a big rush to the emergency room if shortness of breath occurs, or if heart rate is climbing, blood pressure is dropping, or chest pain occurs. Heavy bleeding could indicate incomplete abortion or perforation of an organ such as the uterus, cervix, or vagina. You should report to emergency care if you:

- Run a fever over 100.4°F/38°C for over 12 hours, esp. if combined with any of the following:
- Suffer increasing cramping low abdominal pain not relieved by your usual pain control methods
- Have vomiting and diarrhea for over 24 hours
- Pass clots larger than a golf ball
- Have unusual, foul-smelling vaginal discharge

Going to the emergency room or urgent care center for heavy bleeding or other major concerns does not necessarily mean you or anyone else will be in trouble. Doctors are not police. They are very busy and their only job is to help make you well again. In cases of heavy vaginal bleeding, doctors will ask about your LNMP (LMP) and ask that you describe the bleeding and other symptoms such as pain, dizziness, nausea, bloating, etc. Share your LNMP date if asked, focus on sharing symptoms only, and allow them to do their job.

In *The Story of Jane*, Laura Kaplan describes how the Jane Collective in Chicago took no risks, and so did send some clients to the hospital, thus: "Whenever a woman had to go to the hospital, her counselor prepared her. She needed to know that she had a right to treatment, to refuse treatment, and to be fully informed. If she was threatened by hospital personnel or the police questioned her, she did not have to say anything. Because medical authorities presumed the woman's ignorance, the best strategy at the emergency room was to act dumb. It was one way to use the medical profession's prejudices to the benefit of women."

Check in with one another within the first 24 hours, and make contact again a week afterward to make sure everything is still going well. Bleeding should be tapering off. Signs of pregnancy such as nausea, swollen breasts, bloating, constipation, and fatigue should also be fading. You might be one of the only people they can talk to about their experience, so set aside some time in your schedule so they can be heard.

Medicalized Supplies

As you practice and meet more fellow practitioners, you may encounter new instruments or techniques. Use of the following are not described here because they absolutely medicalize menstrual extraction:

- Laminaria are basically little sticks of compressed seaweed which, once inserted into the cervical os, expand to dilate it. Laminaria are used a lot in clinics because passing through the cervix is not always simple. Abortion medications are sometimes also used for this purpose.

- Tenaculum forceps are long slender tongs with a scissor hand grip and tiny claws at the far end. Tenaculum clasp and stabilize the cervix in a way that can make it easier to pass a cannula. However, they can accidentally scrape or tear the cervix and cause risk of infection. They often leave an "incriminating" bite mark on the cervix.

- Long stainless steel cervical dilator rods in various diameters.

- Para-cervical blocks. Get around in circles enough and you may run into someone providing medications similar to lidocaine via needle to the cervix before cannulation.

- Prophylactic ("just in case") doses of oral antibiotic before menstrual extraction[25] are sometimes given to help prevent complications from pre-existing, often asymptomatic infections such as bacterial vaginosis, chlamydia, and gonorrhea

If you are working alongside anyone using these interventions during menstrual extractions or use them yourself, understand that you are now definitely performing medicine. The law could rain down on you quite a bit harder.

Emotional Follow-Through

It is wise to not consider any abortion procedure finished immediately upon the flow of blood. We hope to see a person returned to whole as much as possible after any invasive and potentially emotional experience, and this does not happen instantaneously. There are complications to watch for, physical symptoms to tend to, and the possibility of emotional upset.

---

25 IPAS recommends, if vacuum aspiration performed: Doxycycline 200mg orally, OR Azithromycin 500mg orally, OR Metronidazole 500mg orally ipas.org/resource/recommendations-for-use-of-prophylactic-antibiotics-in-safe-abortion-care-card/

No matter whether we see tears or laughter after an abortion (both totally normal), there may be the opposite the next day, and the next, until assimilation of the experience has occurred. Our confusion over what to think and feel is likely exacerbated by a culture loudly divided over abortion. We have been offered abortions, but yet told it is wrong. One day we have the bastion of Roe v. Wade, the next it has disappeared. Partners who don't want kids but refuse to help with contraception. Parents who nearly drowned us in dolls and want grandchildren but shame us when we become pregnant too young. We think babies are so cute but it just isn't the time. I certainly think babies are so cute and women so awesome that I wanted to be a midwife, but I already knew in my early teens I didn't want children of my own. My three main reasons for not wanting children can be thrown in the mix with the thousands of other perfectly fine reasons.

It isn't easy to choose abortion but remember: it's not a wrong choice, it's your choice. We may go back and forth beating ourselves up for a while. We may grieve the loss of a child. We may be at odds with partners or family in our decision. We may feel like we've momentarily lost our way. Ultimately though, the vast majority of us are relieved after abortion, and eventually a bright future catches up with us.[26] Whatever we feel is OK. We own our bodies and our feelings. We deserve respect. We all deserve happiness. Acknowledge the choice isn't easy, and acknowledge the bravery and strength it takes to make it.

Watch out for hurting and care for it liberally. Oftentimes the best and only thing we can do is lend one another an ear, ask what can be done to help, and give hugs. If you need help, ask for help. Encourage everyone to speak up if they need help. And if you can help, lend yourself to your local self-help group or other pro-choice organization.

Finally, help spread the word such that menstrual extraction becomes common vocabulary and understanding, and the Del-Em and cervix instantly recognizable. Let coat hangers and other sharp pokey objects be removed from the collective conscious' abortion toolbox forever!

---

26   Greene Foster, Diana. *The Turnaway Study: Ten Years, A Thousand Women, and the Consequences of Having—or Being Denied—an Abortion.* Scribner, 2020

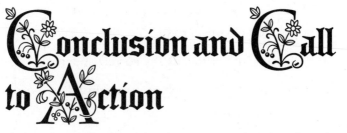

Conclusion and Call to Action

Writing this book immediately after the Dobbs decision was easy; I was animated by grief and rage.

What is difficult is suggesting people leave their comfort zones and possibly put themselves and others at risk. That said, knowledge is power, we are powerful, and this book hopefully powerfully offsets misinformation about abortion care and resets access to our own bodies. When in doubt, please ask for help, and take good care of your badass selves.

This is by no means an exhaustive description of everything there is to know about menstrual extraction. It's a guide to get you acquainted with the method, and yourself. There are substantive obstacles to practicing menstrual extraction safely, such as:

- Understanding female reproductive anatomy and physiology

- Being comfortable with human bodies and ready to help one another

- Sourcing and obtaining the correct supplies

- Finding at least one helper, optimally someone with experience

- Understanding contraindications and risks and being able to decline care

- Anticipating and dealing with surprises and potential complications

- Bravely moving forward in practicing this important skill, despite social and physical discomfort, and accepting that one outcome could be persecution and/or arrest

- Committing to maintain anonymity, privacy and security of all participants while yet attempting to spread the word

We urge those moving forward through these steps to emphasize self-education and acceptance of help, and to re-evaluate the plan whenever something doesn't seem right.

Ideas for Getting Started in Your Area

Start by asking one or two of your close friends if they would like to learn more about their body with you. If any of you is experiencing pelvic pain, unusual vaginal fluids or odors, abnormal periods, difficulty conceiving, or are just curious, it's a great incentive to get started empowering and reassuring yourselves. Study together and normalize pelvic exams between yourselves to the point where it doesn't feel awkward or embarrassing (this usually happens faster than you'd think).

Critique one another, establish work flows and an agreed-upon etiquette, then write down rules for how to proceed when more people are added to the group. Gather supplies, such as lube packets and plastic speculums, and brainstorm how they could be distributed (and normalized). Decide if and at what point you might open the group up further, and maybe each invite another close friend. This can happen fast or slow, but be prepared for your friends to get excited and want to share, and for the group to grow! Some people may decline to join or stop showing up but keep in mind that you have still sown a seed of knowledge and curiosity, which counts as a success.

Continue with monthly living room meetings, where health topics can be discussed, sharing encouraged, and exams practiced when desired. It's best to announce exam days in advance so nobody is surprised. Build expertise and confidence in rapport-building, history-taking, and examination technique. Study your findings and compare notes with your new team. Accept and work with feedback. Soon you or another member may feel confident to outreach and teach.

These meetings are perfectly legitimate and can be broadcast as workshops geared towards groups on social media, including strangers. Inviting medical students to participate is not only a great way to indoctrinate them in empathic care, but also an excellent way to build liaison within the medical community. Of course, ensure that teaching and sharing topics are kept safe for participants, and de-emphasize menstrual extraction in settings where trust is lacking.

You can move into ME training and practice with your closest circle inside the community you have built, and again, after testing the waters, expand your ME circle.

Get out there. Your voice matters, and so many people are ready to hear it!

Notes for the Second Edition

Liberal changes were made after several conversations with Carol Downer. She is not only a powerful voice of self-love and feminism, but a gentle and lucid editor. My deepest thanks to Carol not just for this help, but for a life spent defending people's rights. The book was reorganized to separate menstrual extraction and abortion, and make it more clear that menstrual extraction occurs safely inside supportive and self-correcting self-help networks.

Get in touch: menstrual.extraction@pm.me

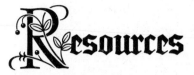esources

National Abortion Federation (NAF) keeps list of active clinics/providers, and provides financial assistance: prochoice.org/patients/naf-hotline/

The most comprehensive directory of trusted (and verified) abortion service providers in the United States: abortionfinder.org/

Center for Reproductive Rights: reproductiverights.org

The Repro Legal Helpline is a free, confidential helpline where you can get legal information or advice about self-managed abortion: reprolegalhelpline.org

Manual Vacuum Aspiration

International Projects Assistance Service (IPAS), providing global MVA tools and education: ipas.org/

IpasU provides free online courses about provision of safe abortion and postabortion care: ipasu.org

Clinical Practice Handbook for Safe Abortion, World Health Organization: ncbi.nlm.nih.gov/books/NBK190097/

Medical Abortion

Help finding and obtaining the Abortion Pill: aidaccess.org and plancpills.org/

Learn more about the Abortion Pill: plannedparenthood.org/learn/abortion/the-abortion-pill

World Health Organization (WHO) recommendations on medical abortion: apps.who.int/iris/bitstream/handle/10665/278968/9789241550406-eng.pdf?ua=1

Using the Abortion Pill in a "Self-Managed, Safe and Supported" manner: abortionpillinfo.org/

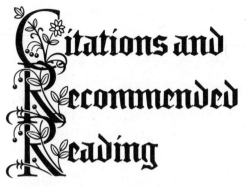

Citations and Recommended Reading

Highly recommended reading is starred.

Bates, CK, Carroll N, Potter J. "The Challenging Pelvic Examination" Journal of General Internal Medicine vol 26, no. 6, June 2011, pp. 651-657 online: ncbi.nlm.nih.gov/pmc/articles/PMC3101979/

*Boston Women's Health Book Collective *Our Bodies, Ourselves.* Simon & Schuster, 1998 – *The one and only, a bible of feminist health, sadly now out of print*

Chalker, R., Downer, C. *A Woman's Book of Choices: Abortion, Menstrual Extraction, RU-486.* Seven Stories Press, 1996

The Doula Project *DIY Doula: Self-Care for Before, During, & After Your Abortion.* Eberhardt

Press, 2016 online: archive.org/details/ DIYDoulaZine/

*Gage, S. When birth control fails: how to abort ourselves safely. Speculum Press, 1979 online:

archive.org/details/DIYabortZine/ – *A seminal dispatch from the Federation of Feminist Women's Health Centers, originally written for Chilean women imprisoned and raped during the Pinochet regime, it became very controversial because it made allowances for the less-than-sterile, DIY conditions these women faced*

*Greene Foster, D. *The Turnaway Study: Ten Years, A Thousand Women, and the Consequences of Having - or Being Denied - an Abortion.* Scribner, 2020 – *Greene Foster describes her compelling longitudinal study showing how abortion changes lives.*

Jeunet, C.M. *Reclaiming Our Ancient Wisdom: Herbal Abortion Procedure and Practice for Midwives and Herbalists* Microcosm Publishing, 2019

Kaufmann, K. *The abortion resource handbook.* Simon & Schuster, 1997

*Lowik, A.J. Trans-Inclusive Abortion Services: A Manual for Providers on Operationalizing

Trans-Inclusive Policies and Practices in an Abortion Setting. Fédération du Québec pour le

planning des naissances, 2018 web. archive.org/web/20210122023137/ womenshealthinwomenshands.com/wp-content/uploads/2018/10/FQPN-Manual-EN-Web.pdf – *Written for Canada, but applicable worldwide.*

Paul, M., Lichtenberg, S., Borgatta, L., Grimes, D., Stubblefield, P. *A clinician's guide to medical and surgical abortion.* Churchill Livingstone, 1999

Presser, Lizzie "Whatever's your darkest question, you can ask me: A secret network of women is working outside the law and the medical establishment to provide safe, cheap home abortions." *The California Sunda Magazine* March 2018 online: story.californiasunday. com/abortion-providers/

Reagan, L.J. *When abortion was a crime: women, medicine, and law in the United States, 1867-1973.* University of California Press, 1997

Sage-Femme Collective *Natural Liberty Rediscovering Self Induced Abortion Methods* Sage-femme! 2008 online: archive.org/details/22321349-natural-liberty-rediscovering-self-induced-abortion-methods

Shotwell, H.G.D. *Empowering the body: The evolution of self-help in the women's health movement.* The University of North Carolina at Greensboro, PhD dissertation, 2016 online: web.archive.org/web/20220716193815/libres.uncg.edu/ir/uncg/f/DudleyShotwell_uncg_0154D_11873.pdf

*Tiamat, U.M. *Herbal Abortion: The Fruit of the Tree of Knowledge* Sage Femme 1994

*Wagner, M. *Born in the USA: How a Broken Maternity System Must Be Fixed to Put Women and Children First.* University of California Press, 2008 – *Friends don't let friends give birth without reading this first.*

Liss-Schultz, N. "Inside the Top-Secret Abortion Underground." *Mother Jones* March/April 2018 online: motherjones.com/crime-justice/2018/02/inside-the-top-secret-abortion-underground

Be the person you want to be and change the world around you at Microcosm.Pub

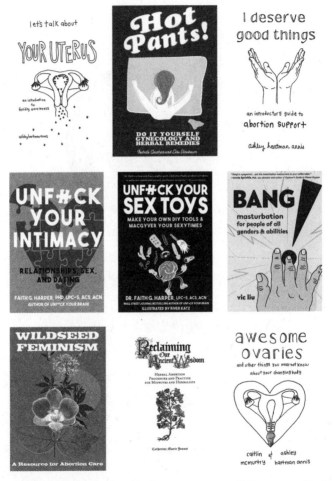

let's talk about

YOUR UTERUS

an introduction to fertility awareness

ashley hartman annis

Hot Pants!

DO IT YOURSELF
GYNECOLOGY AND
HERBAL REMEDIES

I deserve good things

an introductory guide to
abortion support

ashley hartman annis

UNF#CK YOUR INTIMACY

RELATIONSHIPS, SEX, AND DATING

FAITH G. HARPER, PHD, LPC-S, ACS, ACN
AUTHOR OF UNF*CK YOUR BRAIN

UNF#CK YOUR SEX TOYS

MAKE YOUR OWN DIY TOOLS &
MACGYVER YOUR SEXYTIMES

DR. FAITH G. HARPER, LPC-S, ACS, ACN
WALL STREET JOURNAL BESTSELLING AUTHOR OF UNF*CK YOUR BRAIN
ILLUSTRATED BY RIVER KATZ

BANG

masturbation
for people of all
genders & abilities

vic liu

WILDSEED FEMINISM

A Resource for Abortion Care

Reclaiming Our Ancient Wisdom

Herbal Abortion
Procedure and Practice
for Midwives and Herbalists

Catherine Marie Jeunet

awesome ovaries

and other things you may not know
about your changing body

caitlin &   ashley
mcmurtry   hartman annis

More building blocks of care at www.Microcosm.Pub

Subscribe!

For as little as $15/month, you can
support a small, independent publisher
and get every book that we publish—
delivered to your doorstep!

www.Microcosm.Pub/BFF